Essentials of
Gynecologic and Obstetric
Endocrinology

Dedicated
To Fran and the children,
because they care

Essentials of Gynecologic and Obstetric Endocrinology

Habeeb Bacchus, Ph.D., M.D., F.A.C.P.

Associate Professor of Medicine
Loma Linda University School of Medicine;
Associate Chief of Medicine
Consultant in Gynecologic Endocrinology
Associate Clinical Pathologist
Riverside General Hospital

Springer-Science+Business Media, B.V.

Published by
MTP
MEDICAL AND TECHNICAL PUBLISHING CO. LTD.
St. Leonards House
Lancaster, England

First Published by
UNIVERSITY PARK PRESS
Chamber of Commerce Building
Baltimore, Maryland 21202

ISBN 978-0-85200-136-3   ISBN 978-94-011-9834-9 (eBook)
DOI 10.1007/978-94-011-9834-9

Contents

Preface

This book concisely presents the essential information in the field of gynecologic endocrinology. Textual material is extensively supplemented by schemes, tables, and diagrams to elucidate etiologies, pathophysiologic mechanisms, and natural histories of the various clinical disorders in the field. The most timely and up-to-date laboratory procedures and physiologic manipulations for diagnosis are presented. Management rationales based on the definitive diagnostic studies and on knowledge of the natural histories are also presented. Special emphasis is placed on the roles of suprahypothalamic as well as extragonadal and peripheral factors in the pathogenesis of many of the disorders of the menstrual cycle. These include the influence of diseases, altered physiologic states, and drugs—areas which are largely neglected in other presentations of this field.

The material presented is based on courses in gynecologic endocrinology presented at the Loma Linda University School of Medicine and at other institutions over the past several years. Extensive use is made of authoritative reviews in this field, and only highly controversial material is authenticated by specific references.

I am deeply grateful to Mrs. Lucille Innes of the Audiovisual Department at Loma Linda University for the artwork. The loyal secretarial help of Alice Hickman, Carol Guzman, and Robbie Cleek is gratefully acknowledged.

Habeeb Bacchus, Ph.D., M.D., F.A.C.P.

1
Mechanisms of Hormone Actions

Compared with other metabolic active compounds, hormones circulate in extremely low concentrations in the body fluids. Blood levels of peptide hormones normally range from 10^{-10}–10^{-12} M, whereas glucose circulates at the concentration of 10^{-2} M. These low hormone levels, therefore, require special mechanisms for recognition by target cells and for their metabolic activities. Marked organ specificity for actions of hormones are well recognized; for example, the hormone adrenocorticotropin (ACTH) acts on adrenal cortical cells specifically. The product of adrenocortical secretion, cortisol, on the other hand, has several specific targets with special mechanisms to mediate the biologic activity of the hormone. The hormones regulate growth differentiation and metabolic activities of their target tissues. While they do not take part in energy production, hormones are intimately involved in regulation of that process. Actions of most hormones are mediated by two general mechanisms, either through involvement of membrane adenyl cyclase (Sutherland, 1972) or through participation of specific cytosol and receptor molecules (Means and O'Malley, 1972). The detailed mechanisms of actions of insulin and growth hormone actions are not completely clear. Most of the peptide and glycoprotein hormones initiate their actions by activating membrane adenyl cyclase, whereas the steroid hormone actions are mediated by specific cytosol and nuclear receptor proteins. These mechanisms will be summarized below.

HORMONAL ACTIONS PROPAGATED BY RELEASE OF MEMBRANE ADENYL CYCLASE

The release of adenyl cyclase from the inner layer of the cell membrane is a hormone action in many endocrine as well as non-endocrine tissues (Suther-

1

land, 1972; Gill, 1972). Luteinizing hormone (LH) specifically acts on cells of the testes and ovaries to release membrane adenyl cyclase, but there are recent data to implicate its action on certain androgen- or estrogen-producing cells in the adrenal cortex. The hormone regulates growth and replication of cells of the follicle of the ovary as well as the differentiated function, steroidogenesis, in these cells.

The initial event in the action of the hormone is a calcium-independent stereospecific binding of LH to the outer cell membrane of the ovarian (granulosa-thecal) cells. This step initiates the release of adenyl cyclase from the inner membrane layer by a calcium-dependent process, the influx of calcium being activated by the initial membrane receptor binding. Studies with other tissues have shown that this type of receptor binding is undoubtedly related to specific molecular structure at the binding site. Alterations of this structure by disease (e.g., neoplasm) affect the binding affinity and may depress the specificy of their actions. For example, the lys-lys-arg-arg sequence is especially important in the binding of ACTH on the adrenal cell. Adrenal tumor-line cells apparently lose this amino acid configuration and receptor specificity, thereby permitting binding by thyroid-stimulating hormone (TSH), follicle-stimulating hormone (FSH), and LH to this site.

The release of membrane adenyl cyclase initiates a series of intracellular events depicted in figure 1.1. Cyclic adenosine monophosphate is released from adenosine triphosphate (ATP) by the adenyl cyclase enzyme by a process not requiring protein synthesis. This step is extremely efficient and the process of magnification permits the release of several molecules of cAMP per molecule of LH. The cAMP functions as a second messenger mediating LH action. The released cAMP is firmly and specifically bound to a receptor protein, but certain closely related analogs with the $3',5'$ cyclic ring such as guanosine monophosphate and inosine monophosphate may weakly compete for the receptor site. The receptor protein is localized in the cytosol and the endoplasmic reticulum of the cell. Formation of the cAMP-receptor complex permits the release of a protein kinase. The cAMP receptor complex is resistant to the enzyme phosphodiesterase but the enzyme readily degrades cAMP. These steps outlined above describe the major action of cAMP in mammalian tissues, namely the regulation of a cAMP-dependent kinase. The protein kinase transfers the γ phosphate of ATP to serine and threonine residues in a variety of substrate proteins. The cAMP receptor protein kinase contains a regulatory receptor and a catalytic kinase unit which is inhibited by the cAMP receptor. Dissociation of the receptor catalytic complex, which is located in the endoplasmic reticulum, occurs when cAMP displaces the kinase from the receptor as follows:

Receptor − kinase + cAMP → kinase + receptor − cAMP

The free kinase is the fully activated form and is no longer responsive to

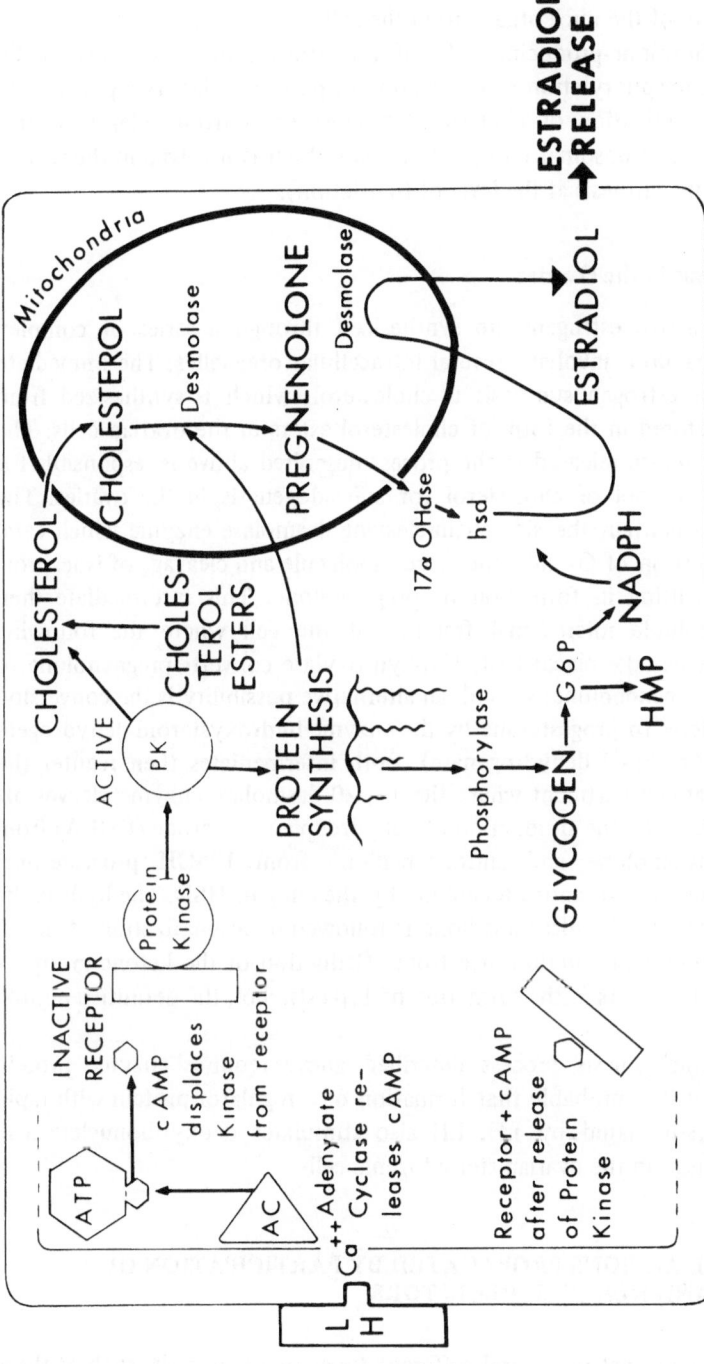

Figure 1.1. Mechanism of action of a prototype peptide hormone. The action of luteinizing hormone (LH) on a steroidogenic cell of the ovarian follicle is depicted. The action of the tropic hormone on the outer cell-membrane is not calcium-dependent, but the release of adenyl cyclase from the inner membrane is. Adenyl cyclase releases cyclic adenosine monophosphate (cAMP) from adenosine triphosphate (ATP). The cAMP displaces protein kinase from the receptor. Protein kinase (PK) then activates several steps as depicted, with eventual production of estradiol.

cAMP. Similar cAMP-dependent kinases are known in several cellular systems, and it is probable that the receptor-cAMP complex may serve to maintain a protected pool of the nucleotide within the cell.

In the hormone-producing cells of the ovaries, the kinase eventually permits the phosphorylation and activation of phosphorylase (via phosphorylase kinase), activation of cholesterol esterase (permitting release of free cholesterol), and ribosomal phosphorylation (which is involved in the regulation of protein synthesis at the level of translation).

Steroidogenesis in the Ovaries

Biologically active estrogens are synthesized through a series of complex enzymatic reactions involving several intracellular organelles. The immediate precursor for estrogen synthesis is cholesterol, which is synthesized from acetate and stored in the form of cholesterol esters in the ovarian cells. The cholesterol esterase released in the process described above is responsible for provision of a pool of cholesterol for steroidogenesis in the ovaries. The mitochondria contain the side chain-cleaving desmolase enzyme which catalyzes the insertion of O_2 into the stored molecule and cleavage of isocaproic aldehyde, resulting in formation of pregnenolone. This intermediate then enters the soluble microsomal fraction of the cell where the following enzymatic steps take place: first, 17α-hydroxylase converts pregnenolone to 17α-hydroxypregnenolone; second, an alternative possibility is the conversion of pregnenolone to progesterone by the enzyme hydroxysteroid dehydrogenase (HSD), Δ^5, 3β-ol dehydrogenase). Both intermediates then reenter the mitochondrial compartment where the 17, 20 desmolase enzyme cleaves off the side chain with the production of dehydroepiandrosterone (DHEA) from 17α-OH pregnenolone and androstenedione from 17αOH progesterone. DHEA is converted to androstenedione by the enzyme HSD. The hydroxylation of carbon 19 of androstenedione is followed by aromatization of ring A with the resultant production of estrone. Reduction of the ketone group of estrone at C 17 results in the formation of 17β-estradiol, the definitive natural estrogen.

The steroidogenesis process described above requires enzyme protein synthesis, and it is probable that formation of a regulator protein with rapid turnover is stimulated by LH. LH also stimulates deoxyribonucleic acid (DNA) synthesis in the ovarian steroidogenic cells.

HORMONAL ACTIONS PROPAGATED BY PARTICIPATION OF CYTOSOL AND NUCLEAR RECEPTORS

Steroid hormones act on several different types of tissue cells, such as those in the liver, kidneys, and adipose tissues, essentially by similar steps (Means

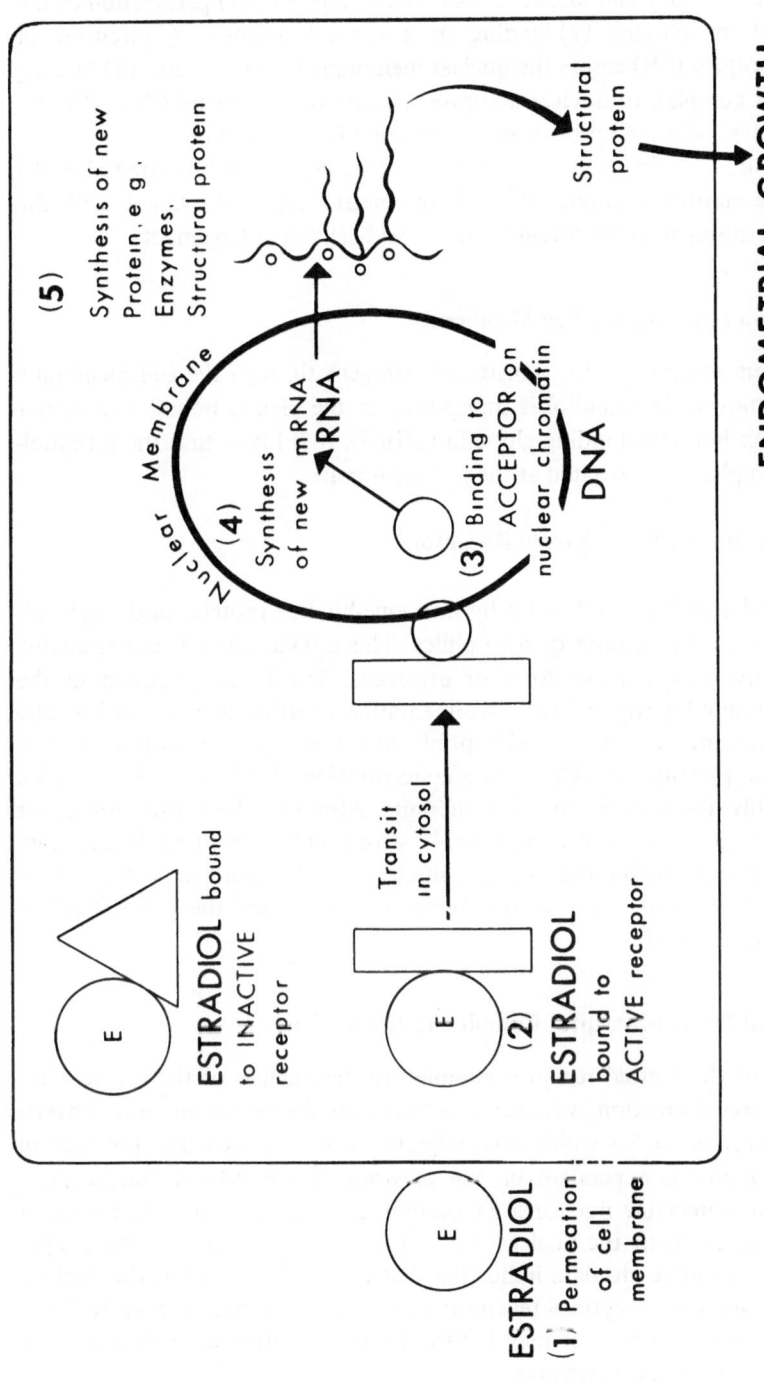

Figure 1.2. Mechanisms of action of a prototype steroid hormone. The action of estradiol on an endometrial cell is depicted. The initial active protein receptor in the cytosol is crucial. Entrance of the steroid-receptor complex into the nuclear compartment permits attachment of the steroid to nuclear chromatin. New enzyme and structural protein synthesis results.

and O'Malley, 1972; Samuels and Tomkins, 1970; Jensen and DeSombre, 1973; and O'Malley and Means, 1974). These steps are: (1) permeation of the target cell membrane; (2) binding to a cytosol receptor; (3) transfer of steroid-receptor (SR) across the nuclear membrane to the nucleus; (4) binding of the SR complex to nuclear acceptor to acceptor chromatin DNA; (5) synthesis of new DNA; (6) protein synthesis; and (7) cell function.

In figure 1.2, the processes stated above are depicted with estradiol as the prototype steroid hormone and the endometrial cell as the target, with the process resulting in new protein synthesis and cellular enlargement.

Permeation of the Target Cell Membrane

The factors responsible for transfer of estrogens through the cell membrane are not known. As estradiol is transported in the plasma bound to a carrier protein sex hormone-binding globulin (SHBG), it is likely that the estradiol-SHBG complex is dissociated at the cell membrane.

Binding to Intracellular Cytosol Receptor

Unchanged estradiol is taken up by hormone-binding proteins in the cytosol, termed estrogen-receptors or estrophiles. This uptake phase is not saturable even at hyperphysiologic doses of estrogens. The binding protein in the cytosol is now known to have a sedimentation coefficient of about 8 s. The estrogen-receptor complex is susceptible to intracellular electrolyte changes and, in the presence of KCl above a concentration of 0.2 M, the 8 s complex is reversibly dissociated into 4 s subunits. Although the estrogen-receptor binding is noncovalent, it is remarkably strong and resistant to dissociation. In some steroid target tissues, *e.g.,* glucocorticoid-dependent cells, at least two conformational types of receptors, one active and the other inactive, have been described.

Transfer of Steroid-Receptor Complex to the Nucleus

Transfer of the steroid receptor complex to the nucleus of the cell requires receptor transformation, whereas a temperature-dependent process converts the 4 s protein to 5 s which then migrates to the nucleus. The presence of nuclear binding is dependent on the presence of the cytosol receptor, and there is no detectable nuclear 5 s protein in cells not exposed to estrogen. As estradiol reacts with the nuclear receptor, there is a decrease of the cytosol receptor, and there are data indicating that estradiol, on leaving the nucleus, may encounter more cytosol receptors and repeat the interaction cycle. Thus, each molecule of estradiol may induce the translocation of several receptor moieties to the nuclear receptor.

Binding of the Estradiol-Receptor (ER) Complex to Nuclear Acceptor (NAc)

The intranuclear binding of the ER involves a two step reaction, first a high affinity reaction between a receptor subunit and chromatin DNA and, second, a high affinity reaction between a specific subunit of the intact native protein and nonhistone (acidic) acceptor proteins.

Synthesis of New Messenger Ribonucleic Acid (mRNA)

Estradiol induction of protein synthesis involves enhancement of precursor incorporation into ribosomal mRNA by a mechanism involving increased nucleolar RNA polymerase activity. The specificity is dependent on the specific activation of mRNA synthesis by the steps described above. It is likely that the ER complex inhibits a repressor gene and, thus, permits activity of a structural gene to stimulate RNA polymerase activity and the resultant release of mRNA. Existence of a post-transcriptional repressor which inhibits translation of specific mRNAs and increased degradation of the messenger is likely, and it is probable that the ER complex inhibits this repressor.

Synthesis of New Proteins by Ribosomes

The synthesis of structural and enzyme proteins in the endometrial cell is directed by the mRNAs released by the above processes. These proteins participate in growth and metabolic activities of the endometrial cells.

REFERENCES

Gill, G. N. 1972. Mechanism of ACTH action. Metabolism 21:571–589.
Jensen, E. V., and E. R. DeSombre. 1973. Estrogen-receptor interaction. Science 182:126–134.
Means, A. R., and B. W. O'Malley. 1972. Mechanism of estrogen action: Early trans-scriptional events. Metabolism 21:357–371.
O'Malley, B. W., and A. R. Means. 1974. Female steroid hormones and target cell nuclei. Science 183:610–620.
Samuels, H. H., and G. M. Tomkins. 1970. Relation of steroid structure to enzyme induction in hepatoma tissue culture cells. J. Molec. Biol. 52:57–74.
Sutherland, E. W. 1972. Studies on the mechanism of hormone action. Science 177:401–408.

2
Hypothalamic-
Pituitary-
Ovarian Axis

The hypothalamic-pituitary system is involved in the control of gonadal development and reproductive rhythmicity (Guillemin, 1967; McCann and Porter, 1969; Frohman, 1973). The gonadotropic hormones, follicle-stimulating hormone and luteinizing hormone, participate in the activation and support of gonadal differentiation and maturation and in the process of hormonal steroidogenesis in the ovaries. Menstrual cyclicity is dependent on the secretion of gonadotropic hormones in adult amounts and sequence. The development of secondary sexual characteristics, as well as the cyclic release of ova, set the stage for conception and implantation. Although the ovaries contain a fund of several hundred thousand follicles at birth, the cyclic release of ova does not commence until about the age of 13 yr. The factors responsible for this latency period are not known. It is related at least in part to the fact that the responsiveness of ovarian tissue to gonadotropins is age dependent and probably mediated by estrogen production by the theca interna (Goldenberg, Recter, and Ross, 1973).

Control of the anterior pituitary cells which secrete the gonadotropic hormones resides in specific nuclei in the hypothalamus. The hypophysiotropic area of the hypothalamus is located in the medial aspect and includes the median eminence (fig. 2.1). Nuclei in this area are responsible for the synthesis and release of several stimulatory and inhibitory neurohormones which are small peptides, the smallest being the tripeptide thyrotropin-releasing factor or hormone (TRF or TRH). The activity of the various hypothalamic nuclei are in turn under control of transducer neurons located in suprahypothalamic areas. In addition, there is an autoregulator "short feedback" loop through which the gonadotropins may regulate their own secretion rate. These neurons exert catecholaminergic or serotoninergic influ-

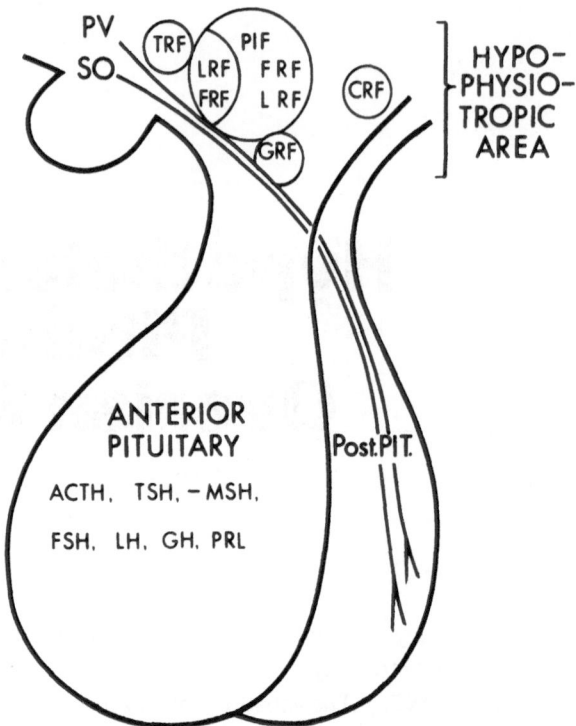

Figure 2.1. Hypophysiotropic area of hypothalamus. The tonic and cyclic centers for release of gonadotropin-releasing hormones are identified. Mapping studies have identified the locations of nuclei releasing the various neurohormones, namely SRF (somatotropin-releasing factor), CRF (corticotropin-releasing factor), TRH (thyrotropin-releasing hormone), PIF (prolactin-inhibitory factor), etc.

ences on the nuclei of the hypophysiotropic areas. Ambient levels of gonadal hormones are involved in the feedback control of release of the hypothalamic neurohormones. This long feedback loop is mainly of the negative feedback type, but there are data which indicate the presence of a positive feedback type of activity also. Yet higher centers exert controlling influences on the axis. The participation of additional suprahypothalamic centers, including the cerebral cortex, the limbic system (amygdala and hippocampus), and the pineal body, has been established.

The existence of gonadotropin-releasing neurohormone(s) has been established. There are data consistent with the view that the release of both FSH and LH is dependent on the secretion of a single gonadotropin-releasing factor (FSH/LH-RH or Gn-RH). Other data suggest separation of LH-releasing and FSH-releasing activities dependent on luteinizing hormone release factor (LRH) and FSH-releasing factor (FSH-RH).

Activity of the suprahypothalamic-hypothalamic-pituitary-ovarian axis is dependent on the integrity of the several nuclei and other responsive cells along the axis, on various factors affecting their responses such as maturation, on factors affecting levels of the circulating hormones such as metabolic degradation and drug effects, as well as temporal factors (fig. 2.2).

MATURATION OF PITUITARY GONADOTROPIN FUNCTION IN FEMALES

Estrogens may exert both a negative and a positive feedback on the pituitary release of the gonadotropic hormone LH. It is at the time of puberty that

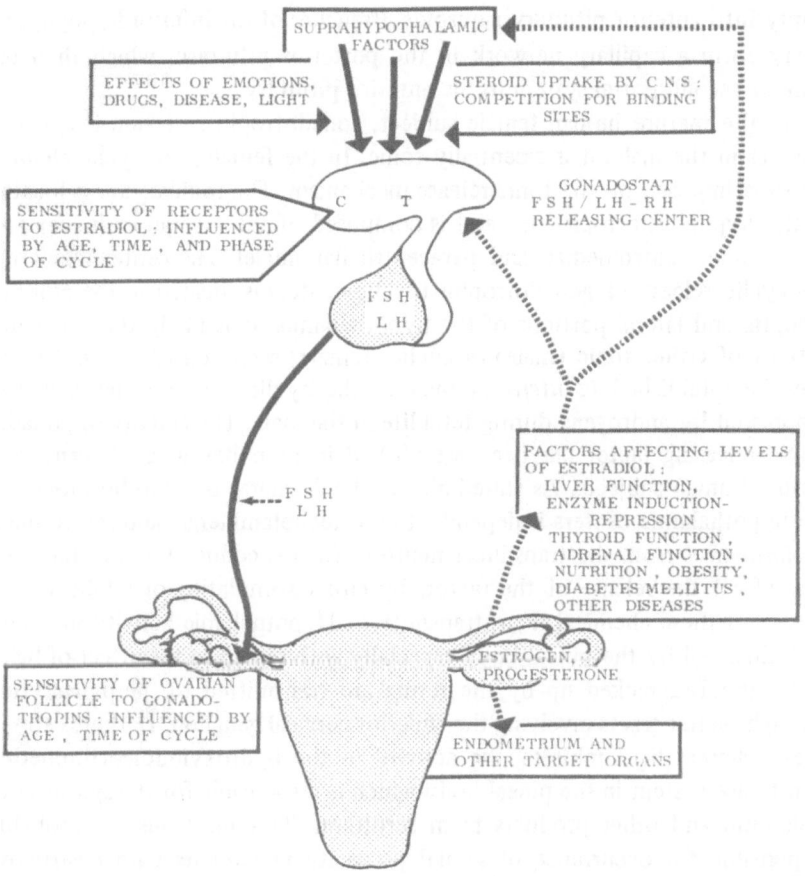

Figure 2.2. Factors affecting the activity of the hypothalamic-pituitary-ovarian axis. The various limbs of the axis are influenced by the various stimuli indicated in the various blocks. Some of these are directly involved in either the hypothalamus, pituitary, or ovaries, whereas others influence the axis indirectly by altering estrogen kinetics or the circulating pool of estrogens and androgens.

estrogens start to elicit the control of LH secretion. Estrogens usually inhibit the release of both FSH and LH (negative feedback), but they may also stimulate the midcycle release of LH which is essential for ovulation (positive feedback). The other ovarian steroid hormone, progesterone, suppresses the secretion of LH and, in conjunction with estrogen, the secretion of FSH.

Suprahypothalamic and hypothalamic areas regulate activity of the anterior pituitary. The neurohormones of the hypothalamus are stored in the median eminence until they are discharged. The neurohormones are transported to the anterior pituitary through a portal system which is derived from the superior hypophyseal artery above and the inferior hypophyseal artery below. A dense capillary network derived from the superior hypophyseal forms portal vessels which traverse the exterior of the pituitary stalk and empty into anterior pituitary sinusoids. Branches of the inferior hypophyseal artery form a capillary network in the posterior pituitary, which then becomes a second portal system to the anterior pituitary.

In the mature human female subject, gonadotropin secretion is cyclical, whereas in the male, it is essentially tonic. In the female, the cyclic changes are superimposed on the tonic release mechanism. The tonic center is located in the hypophysiotropic area and is composed of the median eminence and the arcuate, ventromedial, and paraventricular nuclei. The center regulating the cyclic release of gonadotropins (cyclic center) is located in the anterior preoptic and lateral portions of the hypothalamus. It is likely that the adult pattern of either tonic (male) or cyclic (female) secretion of gonadotropins may be established *in utero* in man as the cyclic center is permanently suppressed by androgens during fetal life in the male. The activity of gonadotropic releasing factor has been established in prepubertal, adolescent, and mature human subjects. As stated above, the discharge of neurohormones by the hypothalamic centers is dependent on catecholaminergic and serotoninergic influences from the transducer neurons. In this connection, several drugs may affect the release of the factors by either stimulating or inhibiting the release of these chemical neurotransmitters. Hypothalamic activity may also be influenced by the pineal body especially with regard to the effect of light. Light impulses picked up by the retina are transmitted to the pineal body through neural tracts involving the superior cervical ganglion. Darkness stimulates, whereas light inhibits, the activity of the hydroxyindoleorthomethyl transferase system in the pineal body which is responsible for the synthesis of melatonin and other products from serotonin. This mechanism is probably responsible for occurrence of sexual precocity in patients with destructive tumors of the pineal body, and of sexual infantilism in patients with functioning (parenchymatous) tumors of the pineal body. The finding of early menarchial ages of blind girls perhaps contradicts the predicted effect of pineal involvement in this process.

It is likely that each component of the pathways which control sexual development in the female, including the end-organs, the gonads, the pituitary, the hypothalamus, and the various suprahypothalamic centers, is capable of adult activity by months or years before the usual age of puberty. The factors responsible for triggering the changes associated with puberty are not fully understood. There are data indicating that the entire axis may already be functional in the fetal and prepubertal states, suggesting that puberty really represents a gradual and continuous progression of a system which started *in utero*. Figure 2.3 presents the changes in the axis at various stages of development.

Undoubtedly, activity of the entire system will depend not only on the release of the various neurohormones and hormones, and their feedback regulation, but also on responsiveness of the particular target tissues. Peripheral metabolic transformation and degradation, time and duration of exposure, as well as levels of exposure, undoubtedly influence the activity of the entire system.

Variations in the sensitivity of the hypothalamic receptor systems may influence the inhibitory and stimulatory effects of gonadal hormones. It is established that this sensitivity of inhibitory influences declines with maturity. The antiestrogenic effects of clomiphene, which are evident in mature subjects (with release of LH and FSH), are not noted in immature children, the adult effect of clomiphene becoming evident in the late stages of puberty. Supporting this concept is the clinical observation that the serum gonadotropins in normal prepubertal subjects and in subjects with gonadal dysgenesis are suppressible with smaller amounts of exogenous estrogens than required in mature individuals. Similarly, the suppressive dose of estrogen increases with age. These phenomena are probably not dependent on chronologic age *per se* in view of the fact that adult sequence and amounts of gonadotropic hormones occur in sexual precocity. It has been suggested that suprahypotha-

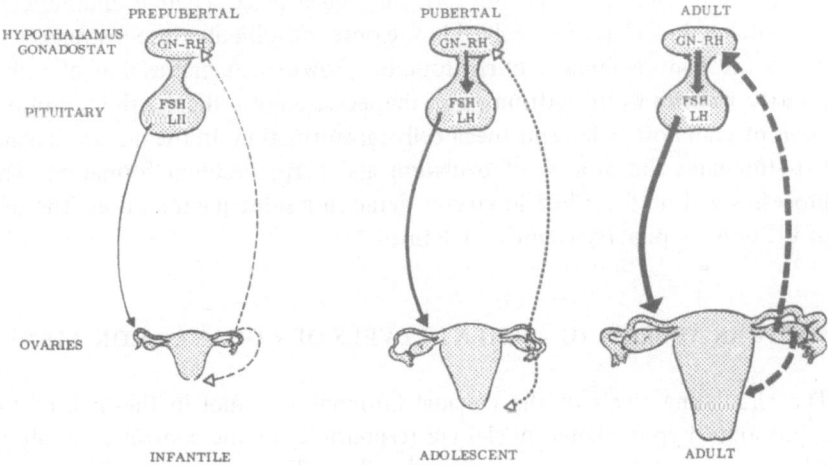

Figure 2.3. Maturation of the hypothalamic-pituitary-ovarian axis.

lamic activity may be responsible for the enhanced inhibitory sensitivity of the hypothalamus to estrogens; inhibition of hypothalamic hypophysiotropic activity by the amygdala has been shown (Schiaffini and Martini, 1972).

In summary, this aspect of hypothalamic-pituitary function is undoubtedly influenced by several factors at different levels of the axis. The decreased sensitivity of the inhibitory hypothalamic centers to estrogens declines progressively with aging. Therefore, relatively larger amounts of gonadotropins are secreted until increased levels of estrogens break through the diminished inhibitory activity of the hypophysiotropic areas. Undoubtedly, there is a continuous process of equilibration until the adult relationship is established.

Chemical and biologic properties of the various pituitary hormones are summarized later in this chapter. Measurable levels of FSH have been found in the urine of girls between the ages of 4.75 and 10.5 yr (Root, 1973); and the urinary excretion of FSH increases between 5–8 yr. In the adult, cyclic variations in FSH correlated with the menstrual cycle. Cyclic changes may also be seen in premenarchial and early postmenarchial girls. LH levels in the urine may be elevated between 3–6 mo of age, with a significant decrease to low levels until age of 6 yr. Serum LH levels increase after 8 yr of age and during the earliest phases of puberty.

OVARIAN RESPONSE TO GONADOTROPINS

Recent experimental data demonstrate that the onset of ovarian responsiveness to exogenous gonadotropins is mediated by estrogen produced by the theca interna (Goldenberg et al., 1973). Since this layer secretes estrogen, it is suggested that the further development of the ovarian follicle is estrogen dependent. Estrogen secreted by the theca interna stimulates granulosa cell proliferation after which antrum formation takes place. There is undoubtedly a time-related mechanism involved in the onset of follicular responsiveness.

In the mature female, FSH promotes growth and maturation of a few primary follicles to the antrum stage, the secretion of follicular fluid, proliferation of granulosa cells, and theca cell transformation. In the mature female, LH stimulates the process of ovulation and corpus luteum formation. The processes will be described in greater detail in a subsequent section. The role of LH prior to puberty is not well defined.

FACTORS AFFECTING AMBIENT LEVELS OF GONADAL HORMONES

The circulating levels of the gonadal hormone estradiol in the area of the appropriate hypothalamic nuclei are responsible for the control of pituitary release of gonadotropic hormones under the influence of hypothalamic neurohormones (LRH, FRH). Factors which alter the levels of 17β-estradiol, therefore, affect the operation of the hypothalamic-pituitary-ovarian axis. Several such factors are now known and include liver function, thyroid function, exogenous obesity, dietary changes, disease states, and drug effects (fig. 2.2).

Effect of Liver Function

The conversion of estradiol to the less active compound, estriol, takes place in the liver. There are considerable data that the degradation of 17β-estradiol is decreased in hepatocellular disease (Chopra, Tulchinsky, and Greenway, 1973). The resultant undegraded estradiol suppresses the cyclic release of FSH and LH. A similar defect in estradiol inactivation in liver disease in males is implicated in pathogenesis of gynecomastia (Chopra et al., 1973). Milder degrees of liver disease, as in fatty metamorphosis of the liver, may be associated with errors in estrogen degradation and may be responsible for secondary amenorrhea. This disorder is often reversible with appropriate management of the liver disorder. Among the causes of fatty metamorphosis known to be associated with menstrual irregularities are exogenous obesity and drug ingestion. Febrile states may also affect menstrual cyclicity presumably by affecting the degradation of the gonadal hormones (fig. 2.2).

Several studies reveal that the hepatic degradation of estrogens, as well as of other steroids, is altered by changes in thyroid function. Spontaneous hyperthyroidism and chronic excess of exogenous thyroid hormones are known to be causes of oligomenorrhea, amenorrhea, and anovulation. Changes in menstrual pattern are also seen in hypothyroidism presumably as a reflection of alterations in degradation of gonadal hormones by the liver and other tissues.

Steroid Conversion in the Central Nervous System

Experimental data reveal that several parts of the central nervous system are active in steroid degradation. Based on the 5α-reductase and 20α-hydroxysteroid dehydrogenase activities of the brain, pituitary, and hypothalamus, a concept has evolved regarding the participation of the central nervous system in regulation of the hypothalamic centers. The 5α-reduction of testosterone decreases the availability of this substrate for the 5α-reductase, and estrogens have been shown to enhance this 5α-reduction of progesterone. Based on these data, Herman, Heinrichs, and Tabei, 1973 speculate that these activities in the central nervous system may well be involved in the feedback regulation of gonadotropin secretion.

In summary, regulation of the hypothalamic-pituitary-ovarian axis is dependent on several factors at several levels of the circuit. Among these are:

(1) sensitivity to negative feedback regulation; (2) sensitivity to positive feedback regulation; (3) responsiveness of target cells based on age- or time-related phenomena; and (4) dependence of the circulating levels of gonadal hormones which are affected by peripheral metabolism in the liver, central nervous system, and other tissues.

HYPOTHALAMIC-PITUITARY CONTROL OF OTHER ENDOCRINE FUNCTIONS

Regulation of ovarian activity by the hypothalamic-pituitary axis has been described in some detail in the preceding section. Similar considerations generally apply in discussing regulation of other target endocrine organs, *e.g.*, thyroid, adrenals, and testes, and regulation of metabolic activities in muscles, adipose cells, and other tissues by growth hormone. The presence of several hypothalamic releasing and inhibitory neurohormones is now established. Control of the nuclei releasing these hormones resides in the activities of transducer neurones which operate through serotoninergic or catecholaminergic pathways. At this level, various drugs which affect synthesis or degradation of these amines may influence activities of the hypothalamic nuclei. Mapping studies have shown the locations of the various hypophysiotropic nuclei in the hypothalamus (fig. 2.1). It is noted that control of growth hormone release is regulated by a nucleus in the ventral aspect of the hypothalamus through the releasing hormone SRF. The site of release of somatotropin release inhibiting factor (SRIF or somatostatin) is located in close apposition. The CRF nucleus which regulates release of adrenocorticotropin (ACTH) by the hypothalamus is located in the posterior aspect of the hypothalamus close to the mamillary bodies. The nucleus for cyclic (surge) release of gonadotropin-stimulating factor(s) is located in the anterior aspect of the hypothalamus, and the nucleus controlling basal secretion of the gonadotropins (the tonic area) is located just posterior to the cyclic nucleus. Thyrotropic releasing hormone (TRH) is secreted by a nucleus located in an anterior aspect of the hypothalamus just above the supraoptic and paraventricular nuclei. It is of interest that this factor may well function as a prolactin-releasing hormone also. Other neurohormones released from the hypothalamus include prolactin inhibitory factor (PIF) and the melanocyte-stimulating hormone (MSH)-inhibiting factors (MIF).

Regulation of the Hypothalamic Nuclei

Release of the corticotropin-releasing factor (CRF) neurohormone from the hypothalamus is inhibited by ambient levels of cortisol. The mechanism of this negative feedback control is not yet clear. The release of ACTH by

Table 2.1. Pharmacologic Effects on Hypothalamic Neurophormone Secretion

Hypothalamic neurohormones	Increased by	Decreased by
Cortocotropin-releasing factor (CRF)	Reserpine (transient), amphetamines, endotoxin	Phenothiazines, cortisol
Thyrotropin-releasing hormone (TRH)	?	T_4, T_3
Gonadotropin-releasing hormone (GnRH; FSH/LH-RH)	Dopamine, L-dopa, estrogens (at certain levels)	Serotonin, melatonin (?), estrogens
Prolactin inhibitory factor (PIF)	L-dopa	Reserpine, phenothiazines, α-methyl dopa
Somatotropin-releasing factor (SRF)	Amphetamines, dopamine, L-dopa	Reserpine, phenothiazines, imipramine, progesterone
Somatotropin release inhibitory factor (SRIF; Somatostatin)	?	?

corticotrope cells of the anterior pituitary is stimulated by CRF. The ambient levels of cortisol do not affect the responsiveness of the pituitary to CRF. In contrast, the response of the pituitary to TRF is altered by the ambient levels of thyroid hormones; the effect of TRF is blocked by high circulating levels of T_3 or T_4. The control of SRF and somatostatin is related to the circulating levels of amino acid and glucose, but the details of the regulation are not completely clear. Control and regulation of the hypothalamic-pituitary-ovarian axis have been discussed in the preceding section.

The various factors which affect the operation of the circuitry which controls the pituitary gonadal axis undoubtedly influence the operations of the other axes considered. For example, it is well known that the pituitary-adrenal relationships are altered in liver disease, by drugs, and in various nutritional states, which may all operate by altering the distribution and degradation of cortisol. In all of the axes described above, suprahypophysial factors may supersede the lower controlling mechanisms discussed. The effects of pharmacologic agents on release of the hypothalamic neuro-hormones are presented in table 2.1.

REFERENCES

Chopra, I. J., D. Tulchinsky, and F. Greenway. 1973. Alterations in circulating testosterone, dehydrotestosterone, estradiol, and gonadotropins in men with hepatic cirrhosis. Clin. Res. 31:200.

Frohman, L. A. 1973. Clinical neuropharmacology of hypothalamic releasing factors. New England J. Med. 286:1391–1397.

Goldenberg, R. L., E. O. Recter, and G. T. Ross. 1973. Follicle response to exogenous gonadotropins: an estrogen-mediated phenomenon. Fertil. & Steril. 24:121–125.

Guillemin, R. 1967. The adenohypophysis and its hypothalamic control. Ann. Rev. Physiol. 29:313–348.

Hermann, W. L., W. L. Heinrichs, and T. Tabei. 1973. Peripheral control of hormone metabolism. Am. J. Obst. & Gynec. 117:679–688.

McCann, S. M., and J. C. Porter. 1969. Hypothalamic pituitary stimulating and inhibiting hormones. Physiol. Rev. 49:240–248.

Root, A. W. 1973. Endocrinology of puberty. J. Pediat. 83:1–19.

Schiaffini, O., and L. Martini. 1972. The amygdala and the control of gonadotropin secretion. Acta Endocrinol. 70:209–219.

3

The Anterior Pituitary Gland

The anterior pituitary gland (adenohypophysis) influences a variety of biologic processes through the secretion and release of polypeptide and glycoprotein hormones (Harris and Donovan, 1966; McCann and Porter, 1969). Body growth is regulated through the synthesis and release of growth hormone (somatotropic hormone, STH), while the structure and activity of several other endocrine glands are regulated by the secretion of various tropic hormones by the anterior pituitary. The gland is derived from ectodermal cells (Rathke's pouch) in the roof of the primitive oral cavity. After migration of these cells upward, and separation from the oral cavity by mesoderm, the cells eventually assume a position anterior to the neurohypophysis. The pituitary gland (anterior hypophysis and neurohypophysis) weighs approximately 500 mg in the normal adult male, and, in pregnant women, may increase to 1 g. The adenohypophysis accounts for approximately 75% of the entire pituitary size. The pituitary gland rests in the sella turcica, a bony structure which surrounds the gland on all sides except the superior surface. The anterior pituitary is supplied by a system of portal veins from a capillary network around the median eminence and the neural stalk (Harris and Donovan, 1966). Within the gland, the portal system divides into sinusoids so that the cells are separated from blood by the endothelium and perisinusoidal space (Harris and Donovan, 1966).

CONTROL OF THE ANTERIOR PITUITARY GLAND

Several stimulatory and inhibitory factors (correctly termed hypothalamic neurohormones) are transported by the portal blood supply to the pituitary gland. The stimulatory hormones include somatotropin-releasing factor (SRF), FSH, and LH-releasing hormone (FSH/LH-RH, or gonadotropin-releasing hormone, GnRH), TRH (thyrotropin-releasing hormone), and CRF (corticotropin-releasing factor). There are some data suggesting probable non-identity of FSH-RH and LH-RH. The inhibitory neurohormones are PIF, MIF, and SRIF or Somatostatin. Suggestions of existence of inhibitory factors corresponding to each of the stimulating factors listed above have not been definitively proved. The various specific secretory cells of the anterior pituitary are under immediate control by the hypothalamic neurohormones. These neurohormones are formed at axonal terminals of tracts which ultimately respond to circulating levels of hormones produced by the target glands, to various metabolic stimuli, e.g., amino acids, and to higher neutral control. These higher neural stimuli may supersede the usual negative feedback circuit.

HORMONES PRODUCED BY THE ANTERIOR PITUITARY GLAND

The anterior pituitary gland is composed of several types of cells which have been characterized by staining and immunofluorescent techniques, different cell types presumably secreting specific hormones. The general groups of cells include the acidophilic cells which secrete growth hormone (GH) and prolactin and the basophilic cells which secrete TSH, FSH, LH, and ACTH. Chromophobe cells may also participate in the secretion of the pituitary hormones.

ACTH, the melanocyte-stimulating hormones (α-MSH, β-MSH), GH, and prolactin possess protein or polypeptide structures, whereas TSH, LH, and FSH are glycoproteins. The tropic hormones, TSH, ACTH, LH, and FSH, maintain the structure and biologic activities of specific target endocrine glands. GH affects several biochemical reactions. ACTH, TSH, and LH increase the activity of adenyl cyclase in the cell membranes of the adrenal cortex, thyroid, and ovary respectively, accelerating the formation of cyclic adenosine, $3'5'$-monophosphate (cAMP) from ATP. Cyclic AMP serves as the intracellular mediator of the action of these hormones.

Growth Hormone

Growth hormone (GH, HGH) (Li, Liu, and Dixon, 1966) is a single chain polypeptide composed of 188 amino acids and has a molecular weight of 21,500. The molecule has an intrachain disulfide bond which forms a ring structure. Because of species differences in immunologic activity, as well as in biologic activity, only primate GH has significant biologic activity in man. GH influences several biochemical mechanisms such as stimulation of protein synthesis, intracellular transport of amino acids, and ribosomal protein synthesis. Intracellular lipolysis is stimulated by the hormone leading to increased plasma free fatty acids and enhancement of fatty acid oxidation and ketogenesis. GH affects carbohydrate metabolism by decreasing the response to insulin, decreasing lipogenesis, and functioning as a diabetogenic hormone in certain species. GH also stimulates collagen synthesis, increases intestinal absorption of calcium, and induces hypercalcemia, sodium, and phosphate retention as well as increasing serum alkaline phosphatase.

GH may require further transformation before becoming effective in growth stimulation. It is suggested that renal uptake of the hormone may be required for its activation. The ability of somatomedin (sulfation factor) to stimulate growth in the absence of GH has been proved (Daughaday, 1971). It is likely that GH (or other hormones) may precede or stimulate the production of somatomedin, which is one of the steps in the process of growth stimulation.

It is estimated that the human pituitary contains 5–10 mg of GH per gland. Normal individuals in the fasting and resting state have a plasma GH concentration of less than 5 mg/ml, with biologic half-life of 20 min. GH levels in the plasma are increased by exercise, hypoglycemia, and infusion or ingestion of certain amino acids such as arginine and are decreased by hypoglycemia. Pituitary GH secretory activity is best assessed after a challenge by one of the above stimuli. These will be discussed later.

Prolactin

Prolactin is a polypeptide hormone with a molecular weight of 23,000 and containing an intrachain disulfide bond. Specific lactotrope cells in the pituitary gland have been identified. Secretion of this hormone is increased by the hypothalamic neurohormone TRH and is suppressed by PIF from the hypothalamus. Several physiologic states, including stress, pregnancy, and anesthesia, and disease states such as chromophobe tumors of the pituitary, as well as several pharmocologic agents, affect the secretion of this hormone (Fourniers, Desjardins, and Friesen, 1974). These are discussed in more detail in Chapter 7. The biologic actions of this hormone include a role in the growth and development of the breast and in lactation. These actions are dependent on the presence of GH, cortisol, thyroid hormone, and progesterone. The mammotropic and lactogenic actions of this hormone have been employed for biologic assays. The hormone is now quantitated by radioimmunoassay methods.

Follicle-Stimulating Hormone

Follicle-stimulating hormone has a glycoprotein structure and an estimated molecular weight of 29,000. Its biologic activity is confined to the gonads, stimulating maturation of the ovarian follicle in the female and increasing the growth of seminiferous tubules and the process of spematogenesis in the male. FSH administration in women is followed by increased levels of urinary estrogens and pregnanediol. FSH extracted from human postmenopausal urine has been employed for induction of ovulation and pregnancy in patients with ovulatory failure, with a high incidence of multiple births. The secretion of FSH by the pituitary is inhibited by estrogens; conversely, in estrogen deficiency, *e.g.*, hypogonadism, there are increased levels of FSH in the urine.

Luteinizing Hormone

Luteinizing hormone is a glycoprotein hormone with an approximate molecular weight of 30,000. This hormone precipitates release of the ovum from the fully developed follicle. It also activates membrane adenyl cyclase, thus releasing cyclic AMP which functions as the intracellular mediator of the steroidogenic action of LH in the follicle and in the corpus luteum. In the male, LH (also called interstitial cell stimulating hormone, ICSH) stimulates the production of testosterone by the interstitial cells of the testis. In prepubertal children, the level of LH measured by radioimmunoassay is 0.5 ng/ml. At puberty in males, the levels reach 0.7 ng/ml, increasing up to 1.7 ng/ml in the fourth decade. In females, the postpubertal level is 1.2 ng/ml in the follicular phase and 1.0 ng/ml in the luteal phase of the menstrual cycle. Detailed patterns of plasma LH during the menstrual cycle have been described (Odell, Ross, and Rayford, 1966). The regulation of LH secretion is dependent on the activity of the central nervous system (Everett, 1964). Estrogens inhibit LH release and, conversely, low levels of estrogens as are found in ovarian insufficiency result in increased LH release. However, a positive feedback between estrogens and LH is necessary for the LH spurt before ovulation. In the male, testosterone has been shown to decrease LH levels (Odell, 1968), but this action is mediated by conversion of testosterone to estradiol.

Thyroid-Stimulating Hormone

Thyroid-stimulating hormone is a glycoprotein hormone containing glucosamine and galactosamine and has an estimated molecular weight of 28,000. TSH increases adenyl cyclase in thyroid tissue and, thus, stimulates the release of cyclic AMP which serves as the intracellular mediator of its action. TSH may also exert an extrathyroidal action on lipolysis in adipose tissue, but the significance of this finding is not clear. TSH increases the thyroidal uptake of ^{131}I, as well as the discharge of thyroid hormone. The release of TSH is determined in large part by the circulating level of thyroid hormone by a negative feedback circuit in which hypothalamic TRH plays a role. However, this role is superseded by the thyroid-pituitary feedback system. By radioimmunoassay procedures (Utiger, 1965), it has been estimated that TSH levels in human plasma range from 0–10 μU/ml, with marked elevations in patients with hypothyroidism and low to undetectable levels in primary hyperthyroid states.

Adrenocorticotropic Hormone

Adrenocorticotropic hormone is a single-chained polypeptide made up of 39 amino acids with species differences in amino acids at positions 25 and 33. The peptide of amino acids 1 through 24 exerts biologic activity of the full ACTH molecule. The major function of ACTH is to maintain the structure and secretory activity of the adrenal cortex. It stimulates the production of cortisol, corticosterone, and 17-ketosteroids (17-KS) by the adrenals by activation of adrenal cell membrane adenyl cyclase which leads to release of cAMP which serves at the intracellular mediator of ACTH action (Gill, 1972). The hormone also exerts a melanocyte-stimulating activity, but increased pigmentation observed in patients with high levels of ACTH is probably due to associated increased MSH levels. There is a circadian pattern in ACTH release, with peak levels occurring at the time of awakening, followed by a steady decline at the time of sleep. The level of ACTH is also dependent on the circulatory levels of cortisol by a negative feedback system mediated by hypothalamic CRF. ACTH depletes the adrenal stores of cholesterol and ascorbic acid, and the latter finding is the basis of a biologic assay for ACTH. The steroidogenic action of ACTH in the hypophysectomized rat's adrenal is another method of biologic assay of ACTH. Employing bioassay methods it was shown that plasma ACTH ranges between 0.1–0.5 μU/100 ml at 6:00 A.M., with undetectable levels at 6:00 P.M. Yalow et al. (1964), employing radioimmunoassay, demonstrated somewhat higher levels of plasma ACTH.

α- and β-Melanocyte-Stimulating Hormones

α-Melanocyte-stimulating hormone (α-MSH) is a polypeptide composed of 13 amino acids, and β-melanocyte-stimulating hormone (β-MSH) is made up of 22 amino acids. There are certain features in these structures which are similar to the amino acid sequence in ACTH. MSH produces dispersion of melanin granules in the skin; this activity has been separated from similar action of ACTH.

ASSESSMENT OF FUNCTIONS OF THE ANTERIOR PITUITARY GLAND

The function of the pituitary gonadal axis is influenced by the various other actions of the gland (Bacchus, 1972; Eddy et al., 1974). It is, therefore, essential that several aspects of its functions are evaluated in the analysis of the various disorders of the pituitary-gonadal axis. The principles and procedures for assessment of pituitary function are presented under headings of individual functions.

Assessment of Pituitary Gonadotropic Functions

These activities of the pituitary are reflected by the functions of the target ovaries in the female. Vaginal cytology and endometrial development are indirect indexes of pituitary effect on the gonads and are discussed in other sections. The differential diagnosis of hypopituitarism from primary gonadal insufficiency requires the determination of plasma or urinary pituitary FSH and LH. In primary gonadal failure, the pituitary gonadotropin levels are higher than normal. These tests are especially useful in the diagnosis of hypopituitarism in the postmenopausal women; in these patients, the increase in urinary gonadotropins associated with the postmenopausal state is absent. In adult women of reproductive ages, normal values for FSH range from 6–30 μU/ml and for LH the normal values are essentially the same. Low values are difficult to interpret, and it is necessary to perform the stimulation tests listed below to assess pituitary gonadotropic responsiveness.

Clomiphene Stimulation Test   In the test, 50 ml of clomiphene is given orally 2 or 3 times daily for 7 days. Plasma is obtained before and after the clomiphene ingestion for FSH and LH determinations. A significant increase ($> 58\%$) in LH after clomiphene is a normal response. The rise in FSH is not as marked. Patients with gonadotropin deficiency fail to show a significant increase in LH.

LRH Stimulation Test   In this test, 50–150 μg FSH/LH RH is injected intravenously and plasma LH and FSH are determined at 0 min, 10 min, 15 min, 30 min, 60 min, 120 min, and 180 min after the injection. The integrity of pituitary gonadotropic activity is reflected by 5- to 10-fold increases in LH and a less marked elevation of FSH at the peak time around the 15- to 30-min interval.

Assessment of Pituitary Adrenocorticotropin Function

Diseases of the pituitary may cause hyperadrenocorticotropinism and hypoadrenocorticotropinism, both of which are manifested clinically by their effects on adrenocortical functions.

Hyperadrenocorticotropinism   Hyperadrenocorticotropinism results in bilateral adrenocortical hyperplasia (Cushing's disease) and hypercortisolemia, as well as increased levels of adrenal 17-KS androgens. Clinical manifestations of hypercortisolemia are due to the effects of the hormone on protein, fat, and carbohydrate metabolism, as well as its effects on blood pressure,

connective tissues, and bone structure. The androgenic effects include virilization and hirsutism in the female. These clinical effects are described in
Chapter 10.

Indirect clinical laboratory effects of hypercortisolemia include an increased blood sugar and impaired glucose tolerance test (GTT), decreased total
eosinophil count in peripheral blood, and an increase in serum Na:K ratio,
but these parameters are not pathognomonic of hypercortisolemia.

Assessment of Pituitary Hyperadrenocorticotropinism These methods
involve quantitiation of adrenocortical steroids or their metabolites after
appropriate physiologic manipulations. These tests are described more fully in
Chapter 10.

In the overnight dexamethasone suppression test, the patient is given 1
mg of dexamethasone orally at 12 midnight, and a plasma cortisol level is
determined on blood drawn at 8:00 A.M. Normal individuals show a plasma
cortisol level of 5 μg/100 ml. Levels of cortisol greater than 10 μg/100 ml are
found in patients with hypercortisolemia due to hyperadrenocorticotropinism, as well as adrenal adenoma, carcinoma, or ectopic ACTH.

Circadian variation of plasma cortisol is lacking in patients with increased
ACTH. Plasma cortisol levels in normal subjects at 8:00 A.M. and at 5:00
P.M. are 5–25 μg/100 ml and 2.5–12.5 μg/100 ml respectively. Patients with
increased ACTH exhibit values of 25 μg or greater at both times.

Basal urinary excretion of 17-hydroxycorticosteroids (17-OHCS) and
17-latogenic steroids (17-KGS) is increased in patients with hypercorticotropinism, adrenal adenoma, adrenal carcinoma, and ectopic ACTH excess.
Urinary 17-KS is also increased in all of the above conditions except adrenal
adenoma. The procedures and the values are described in Chapter 10.

Dexamethasone suppression tests utilizing urinary 17-OHCS (total or
after sequential extraction) or 17-KGS reveal no suppression of urinary
steroids after the low dexamethasone dosage (0.5 mg every 6 hr for 3 days) in
patients with hypercorticotropinism. Suppression occurs after higher doses of
dexamethasone (2 mg 4 times daily for 3 days).

Urinary 17-OHCS (total or fractionated), 17-KGS, or plasma 11-deoxy-
cortisol after metyrapone (oral or intravenous) are significantly increased in
patients with hypercorticotropinism (see Chapter 10).

The biologic assay methods of measuring ACTH levels are not readily
applicable to clinical practice. The radioimmunioassay of ACTH promises to
be quite helpful in diagnosis of pituary-adrenal disorders. In hypercorticotropinism, the levels of ACTH are significantly higher than the normal
0.1–0.5 μU/100 ml.

Hypoadrenocorticotropinism Hypoadrenocorticotropinism   (decreased
ACTH secretion) is manifested clinically by evidence of adrenal insufficiency

described in Chapter 10. Patients with hypoadrenocorticotropinism lack the pigmentary and marked electrolyte disturbances seen in primary adrenal disease.

The best tests to evaluate a defect in ACTH production involve methods of stimulating the release of ACTH. The effects of ACTH release are measured by study of plasma cortisol or urinary corticosteroids. After establishing that the adrenal cortex is responsive (see sections on the intravenous cosyntropin test and the 8-hr ACTH test described in Chapter 10), the following tests may be done.

Vasopressin Stimulation Test   In our experience, this test is very reliable and less cumbersome than any of the other procedures employed. Plasma cortisol increase of 100% or greater after injection of vasopressin (10 units intramuscularly) is reliable evidence of intact pituitary ACTH secretion.

Adrenocorticotropic Hormone Tests   Repeated 8-hr intravenous ACTH tests show incremental increases in urinary 17-KS, 17-KGS, or 17-OHCS in patients with hypoadrenocorticotropinism. A simpler procedure is repetitive cosyntropin stimulation (0.25 mg every hour for 3 doses). Incremental increases are seen in hypoadrenocorticotropin disorders (Bacchus, 1972).

Metyrapone Challenge   The various procedures employing metyrapone challenge are quite reliable for assessment of pituitary ACTH function and are especially helpful in differentiating primary from secondary adrenal insufficiency. The lack of increased levels of plasma 11-deoxycortisol, urinary 17-KGS, 17-OHCS, or THS after metyrapone would be consistent with decreased pituitary ACTH production, provided the adrenal is ascertained to be intact.

Assessment of Pituitary Thyrotropic Function

The target organ effects of TSH on the thyroid are employed in testing for pituitary TSH activity. In the TSH stimulation test, a basal epithyroid ^{131}I uptake increases to normal or supranormal levels after TSH injection (10 units intramuscularly daily for 3 days). In some patients with a long-standing hypopituitarism and marked thyroid involution, no increase is seen after TSH stimulation.

Direct Assessment of Pituitary TSH Function   In primary thyroid insufficiency, the TSH levels are higher than normal ($> 10\ \mu U/ml$); in pituitary insufficiency, the levels are between $0-10\ \mu U/ml$, which is the normal range. It is, therefore, necessary to perform the TRH stimulation test in which the hypothalamic neurohormone TRH is given by intramuscular injection of $50-100\ \mu g$ and plasma. TSH levels are measured before and after the TRH administration. A significant increase in TSH to supranormal levels reflects integrity of pituitary thyrotropic activity. The peak increase in TSH is noted within $20-30$ min after the injection of TRH (Utiger, 1962).

Assessment of Pituitary Prolactin Release

The TRH stimulation test is employed to assess pituitary release of prolactin. Normal individuals show a marked increase in plasma prolactin after TRH injection. (It is well to note the close proximity of the site of TRH production and that of gonadotropin release in the hypophysiotrophic area; see Chapter 8).

Assessment of Growth Hormone Functions

Clinical disorders may involve decreased and excessive GH secretion. These clinical states may be suspected on the basis of the target organ effects of GH.

The clinical features of various pituitary disorders are presented in tables 3.1 and 3.2. In the unihormonal deficiency state involving GH, dwarfism is the resultant clinical condition. In the adult, the major clinical laboratory finding is that of a hypoglycemia which may be symptomatic under conditions of stress. In the child with decreased GH, the most important manifestation is decreased bone age; the epiphyses do not develop at a normal rate, hence, bone age on an X-ray of the wrists, for example, is retarded. Serum phosphate and alkaline phosphatase are often decreased.

Direct Assessment of Decreased Growth Hormone

GH Levels in Hyposomatotropinism Basal fasting serum immunoreactive GH levels of less than 1 ng/ml are found in both types of hyposomatotropinism.

Serum GH Levels after Insulin Hypoglycemia A baseline blood sample is obtained for glucose and GH determinations. The patient is given crystalline insulin by intravenous injection (0.05 units/kg body weight in children, and 0.1 to 0.15 units/kg in adults). Blood samples are obtained at 20, 60, and 90 min after the injection of insulin. An adequate stimulus is a drop of blood sugar to less than 50% of basal value, or below 50 mg/100 ml. Baseline plasma and at least two in the hypoglycemic range are used for GH radioimmunoassay.

Normal subjects show levels of GH 2 to 3 times the basal level of GH, or at least exhibit GH levels of > 10 ng/ml at the hypoglycemic peak. Patients with pituitary insufficiency causing decreased GH, as well as obese individuals, fail to show increased levels of GH. It is suggested that nonresponsiveness of HGH to hypoglycemia should be confirmed by the arginine challenge.

GH Levels after Arginine Infusion A baseline blood sample is obtained for glucose and GH determinations. The patient is given an arginine solution of 0.5 mg/kg body weight by intravenous infusion over a period of 30 min. Blood samples for GH levels are taken at the end of the infusion (30 min) and at 60, 90, and 120 min after the start of the infusion. Normal subjects show increases in the GH levels to 2 to 3 times the basal value. Patients with defective GH secretion fail to show values above 10 ng/ml.

Table 3.1. Clinical Features and Laboratory Diagnostic Studies in Hypopituitarism in Women

Disorder	Etiology or mechanism	Clinical defects	Diagnostic studies
Posthypophysectomy	Surgery or radiation	Due to defect in GH Decreased water diuresis; stress hypoglycemia	Hypoglycemic challenge and plasma GH and cortisol; vaginal cytology; plasma FSH, LH before and after LHRH or clomiphene; T_4, TSH levels combined pituitary challenge (Harsoulis et al., 1974)
		Due to secondary defect in gonads Amenorrhea; vaginal and uterine atrophy	
		Due to secondary defect in adrenal Nausea; vomiting, hypotension; death (early changes at 4–5 days)	
		Due to secondary defect in thyroid Cold intolerance; dry skin, myedema (4–8 wk postoperative)	
Spontaneous panhypopituitarism	Postpartum necrosis of pituitary gland; granulomas; infarction from vascular disease; infection;	Due to defect in GH Stress hypoglycemia	Hypoglycemic challenge and plasma GH and cortisol; vaginal cytology; plasma FSH; LH before and after LHRH or clomiphene; T_4 TSH levels combined pituitary challenge (Harsoulis et al., 1974)

	Hand-Schuller Christian disease; pituitary apoplexy in tumor	Due to defect in gonads Postpartum pituitary necrosis with shock from adrenal insufficiency is earliest manifestation; chronic insufficiency may appear years later	Hypoglycemic challenge and plasma GH and cortisol, vaginal cytology; plasma FSH; LH before and after LHRH or clomiphene; T_4, TSH levels combined pituitary challenge (Harsoulis et al., 1974)
Unihormal; dwarfism	Often unknown etiology; hereditary in a few cases; possible hypothalamic defect	Due to defect in GH Body growth and facial features; immature eruption of secondary teeth late; subclinical hypoglycemia	Bone age; height; plasma GH after insulin or arginine infusion
ACTH deficiency	Possible defect in CRF from hypothalamus	Due to secondary defect in adrenal Nausea; vomiting; weakness; hypotension; decreased axillary and pubic hair	Plasma cortisol or urine 17-OHCS before and after vasopressin or metyropone; ACTH levels
TSH deficiency	Possible defect in hypothalamus	Due to secondary defect in thyroid Cold intolerance; dry skin; myxedema, anemia	TSH levels before and after TRH
Gonadatropin deficiency	X-linked trait; other etiology	Due to secondary defect in gonads Amenorrhea and decreased pubic and axillary hair	Vaginal cytology; endometrial biopsy; plasma FSH and LH before and after LH-R\

Table 3.2. Clinical Features and Laboratory Diagnostic Studies in Hyperpituitarism

Disorder	Etiology	Clinical effects	Diagnostic studies
Gigantism and acromegaly	Acidophilic and chromophobe tumors of pituitary	Prepubertal onset (gigantism): excessive proportional growth, later acral changes; postpubertal (acromegaly): periosteal growth, widening of bones, broad hands, widened fingers with blunted ends; prognathism, teeth widely separated, macroglossia, osteoarthritis, cardiomegaly, cardiomyopathy, congestive heart failure, and diabetes mellitus; hypogonadism is frequent; hirsutism and persistent lactation in some patients	Diabetic-type GTT; bone changes by X-ray; plasma GH, baseline high with failure to suppress after hyperglycemia
Hypersecretion of prolactin	Hypothalamic defect	Chiari-Frommel syndrome; postpuerperal persistent lactation and secondary amenorrhea; vaginal and uterine atrophy	Plasma prolactin
	Pituitary tumors, mainly chromophobe adenoma	Forbes-Albright syndrome; nonpuerperal lactation and amenorrhea; vaginal and uterine atrophy	Plasma prolactin
Hypersecretion of ACTH and MSH	Basophilic adenomas (mainly)	Hypercortisolism, Cushing's syndrome (hypertension, plethora, moon facies, striae, centripetal fat distribution, obesity, and polycythemia); hyperpigmentation, occasional hirsutism and hypertrophy of clitoris	Plasma and urine cortisol and 17-OHCS before and after dexamethasone suppression; ACTH radioimmunoassay; MSH radioimmunoassay
Ectopic ACTH production	Bronchogenic small cell or undifferentiated carcinoma; pancreatic and thymic carcinoma	As above, except for absence of obesity; weight loss may be due to tumor growth	As above ACTH radioimmunoassay (?)

GH Levels after Glucagon   In this test, a similar protocol as in the test directly above is employed. The baseline GH level is compared with those taken 20, 60, and 90 min after the subcutaneous injection of 1.0 mg of glucagon. The criteria for diagnosis are those in the same as those above. This procedure is safter than the assessment after insulin hypoglycemia.

GH Response to Vasopressin Challenge   Baseline plasma, and plasma obtained 30 and 60 min after intramuscular injection of 10 units of vaso-pressin, are followed by a significant rise of GH in normal subjects. Failure to show GH above 10 ng/ml is consistent with hyposomatotropinism.

GH Levels after Physical Exercise   GH levels after vigorous physical exercise, or during deep sleep, are methods employed, especially in pediatric practice, for assessment of hyposomatotropinism.

GH Levels in Plasma after Challenge with Dihydroxyphenylalanine (L-Dopa)   Several studies show that normal individuals exhibit a prompt and significant increase in plasma HGH after oral ingestion of 0.5 g of L-dopa. This test is readily performed on an outpatient basis and is highly reliable (Eddy et al., 1974).

It should be pointed out that the above procedures should not be performed unless the patient is euthyroid, as hypothyroidism will attenuate or obliterate the expected rises in HGH after the various challenges.

Hypersomatotropinism   Hypersomatotropinism (excessive GH) in the prepubertal child results in gigantism, whereas its occurrence after puberty results in acromegaly. Indirect clinical tests consistent with hypersomato-tropinism include a diabetic-type glucose tolerance test, an elevated serum inorganic phosphorus level (without the normal circadian variation), hyper-calciuria, hydroxyprolinemia, and virilization ascribable to increased 17-KS levels.

Direct Assessment of Growth Hormone Excess   These methods involve the determination of GH levels by radioimmunoassay. The basal GH levels in the fasting male subject is 5 ng/ml or less, and a level greater than 5 ng/ml is, therefore, consistent with hypersomatotropinism. In female patients the basal fasting levels may fluctuate widely. It is necessary to conduct a hyper-glycemic challenge before assessing the GH levels.

In male and female patients with acromegaly, there is a less than 50% decrease in plasma immunoreactive GH after infusion of glucose intra-venously. Normal subjects exhibit an almost complete suppression of GH production during the hyperglycemia. Patients with hypersomatotropinism show plasma HGH levels of > 10–300 ng/ml regardless of the level of blood sugar elevation.

The studies are detailed above to present the methods, rationale, and interpretations of the individual tests. It is now recommended that they be replaced by the combined pituitary challenge test (Harsoulis et al., 1974). In this procedure the patients are studied in the fasting state with the test commencing from 9:00 to 10:00 A.M. Regular insulin is administered intravenously (0.05–0.3 units/kg of body weight) and followed immediately by a mixture of 200–500 μg of TRH and 100 μg of FSH/LH-RH in 5 ml of sterile water. Blood samples are obtained at 0, 30, 60, 90, and 120 min after the infusion for quantitation of glucose, growth hormone, and cortisol. TSH, FSH, and LH are determined only at the 0-, 20-, and 60-min intervals. The results obtained in this manner are essentially comparable to those obtained with the separate test procedure. Normal subjects exhibit significant elevations in GH (values reaching > 10 ng/ml by 60 min with mean values around 120 ng/ml), cortisol (values at least 7 μg/100 ml greater than baseline, or a 3- to 4-fold increase by 1 hr), TSH (at least a 4-fold increase by 20 min), FSH (at least a doubling by the 20- to 60-min sampling times), and LH (at least a 2- to 4-fold increase by the 20- to 60-min sampling times). Patients with panhypopituitarism fail to show significant increases in these hormones after the combined challenge.

Clinical Disorders of Anterior Pituitary Function

Clinical patterns in disorders of the anterior pituitary depend on the hormones affected and on the time of onset of the disorder. Because of the multiplicity of anterior pituitary hormones either hyperfunctional or hypofunctional states may be manifested by a combination of disturbances in the target effects of various or isolated (single) pituitary hormones. Etiologies and clinical manifestations of the various clinical disorders are summarized in tables 3.1 and 3.2. Disturbances in the production of the tropic hormones are manifested mainly by clinical and laboratory parameters related to the target organs of the specific tropic hormones. Disturbances in GH secretion are reflected by disturbances in the various tissues effects of GH.

Hypopituitary States Clinical manifestations depend both on age of onset and on the hormones affected.

Hypopituitarism in Childhood The clinical pattern depends on the hormonal functions affected. In panhypopituitarism in childhood, there are several clinical manifestations.

There are manifestations secondary to GH deficiency. Intrauterine growth is not dependent on GH, but subsequent growth is. Therefore, there is marked growth retardation detectable during the first year of life. Serial height-weight measurements, failure of the appearance of certain landmarks at correct times, such as delayed bone age and epiphyseal development, are reliable stigmata of this deficiency. The ratio of upper (crown to pubis) to the lower (pubis to floor) body segments will approach 1:1 in contrast to the infantile 1.7:1.

There are parameters referable to decreased gonadotropins. Pubertal development is retarded. There is lack of female sexual characteristics such as pubarch and thelarche. Epiphyseal closure does not occur and there is no evidence of estrogen effect on the vagina. Linear growth may continue into the third or fourth decade because of lack of epiphyseal closure.

There are clinical parameters referable to lack of TSH. Hypothyroidism tations may not be overt, and may occur only during stress. Occasional hypoglycemia and weakness may occur.

There are clinical parameters referable to lack of TSH. Hypothyroidism may be mild compared with the clinical manifestations in primary hypothyroidism.

Panhypopituitarism in the Adult The manifestations are referable mainly to deficiencies of the tropic hormones since there are no overt clinical manifestations of GH deficiency in the adult. Hypoglycemia may occur under certain stress situations and in the presence of infections. The clinical patterns of this disorder and unihormonal deficiencies are presented in table 3.1.

Treatment of Pituitary Diseases

Diseases of Hyperfunction Most of the hyperpituitary states presented in table 2 are due to tumors. The available methods for therapy of these tumors are conventional radiation, radiation with proton beam, yttrium, radioactive gold implants, and cryosurgery. These methods have been evaluated in several centers, but final data are not available. Conventional radiation has been employed for patients without extrasellar spread, but is probably not completely satisfactory. Proton beam therapy is moderately effective, especially in patients without extrasellar extension; surgery has been performed in patients with local tumor extension with some degree of success. Cryosurgery has been quite successful and has been followed by early decreases of HGH in the acromegalic patients treated. Transsphenoidal implantation with yttrium-90 is also worthwhile, but may be complicated by infection and cerebrospinal fluid rhinorrhea.

Medical management of acromegaly with progesterone and phenothiazines has been attempted, with some evidence of improvement. In the hypothalamic disorder associated with suppression of prolactin inhibitory factor (resulting in inappropriate prolactin release), newer information on pharmacologic agents *e.g.*, L-dopa and others may provide a rationale for therapy (see Chapter 11).

Diseases of Hypofunction Clinical disorders secondary to deficiencies in the tropic hormones are not treated by the pituitary hormones, since all the hormones of the target glands are not available and have not been extensively employed. Replacement therapy includes the following.

Thyroid Hormone Gradual restitution of replacement doses of thyroxin (0.05 mg daily or 15 mg of thyroid extract) is begun. The dosage should be increased gradually until a full replacement dose of 0.15–0.2 mg thyroxin (or

90–120 mg desiccated thyroid) is achieved. The presence of arteriosclerotic heart disease and angina may necessitate slower progression to lower final dose. In myxedema coma, a faster acting preparation triiodothyronine is recommended.

Corticosteroid Replacement Corticosteroid replacement is between 12.5–37.5 mg of cortisone acetate daily. Larger doses may be required in stressful situations. Replacement with a mineralocorticoid is rarely needed in pituitary ACTH deficiency.

Gonadal Hormone Replacement Gonadal hormone replacement in young female patients is achieved with the use of estrogens to prevent osteoporosis and atrophy of the genital organs and vaginal mucosa.

Unihormonal Replacement The rare occurrence of unihormonal deficiency of pituitary tropic hormones is treated by the appropriate target gland product as above.

Treatment of Pituitary Dwarfism   Human growth hormone in doses of 1 mg/day is followed by markedly accelerated growth of up to 3–5 in/yr within the first year. Thereafter, the growth rate is somewhat slower. Occasionally, antibody formation precludes further therapy, but reinstitution after several months may again cause growth. The supply of human growth hormone is limited since it is harvested from cadaver pituitances. Synthetic growth hormone will probably be available soon.

REFERENCES

Bacchus, H. 1972. Endocrine profiles in the clinical laboratory. *In* M. Stafanine (ed.), Progress in Clinical Pathology. Vol. IV, p. 1–101, Grune & Stratton, Inc., New York.

Daughaday, W. H. 1971. Regulation of skeletal growth by sulfation factor. Advances Int. Med. 17:237–263.

Eddy, R. L., P. F. Gilliland, T. D. Ibarra, J. F. McMurry, and J. Q. Thompson. 1974. Human growth hormone release. Comparison of provocative test procedures. Am. J. Med. 56:179–185.

Everett, J. W. 1964. Central neural control of reproductive functions of the adenohypophysis. Physiol. Rev. 44:373–431.

Fournier, P. J. R., P. D. Desjardins, and H. G. Friesen. 1974. Current understanding of human prolactin physiology and its diagnostic and therapeutic implications: A review. Am. J. Obst. & Gynec. 118:337–343.

Gill, G. N. 1972. Mechanism of ACTH action. Metabolism 21:571–589.

Harris, G. W., and B. T. Donovan. 1966. The Pituitary Gland. Vol. 1–3. Univ. California Press, Berkeley.

Harsoulis, P., J. C. Marshall, S. F. Kuku, C. W. Burke, D. K. London, and T. R. Fraser. 1974. Combined test for assessment of anterior pituitary function. Brit. M. J. 4:326–329.

Li, C. H., W. Liu, and J. S. Dixon. 1966. Human pituitary growth hormone XII. The amino acid sequence of the hormone. J. Am. Chem. Soc. 88: 2050–2051.

McCann, S. M., and J. C. Porter. 1969. Hypothalamic pituitary stimulating and inhibiting hormones. Physiol. Rev. 49:240–248.

Odell, W. D. 1968. Gonadotropins: Present concepts in the human. California Med. 109:467–485.

Odell, W. D., G. T. Ross, and P. L. Rayford. 1966. Radioimmunoassay for human luteinizing hormone. Metabolism 15:287–289.

Utiger, R. D. 1965. Radioimmunoassay of human plasma thyrotropin. J. Clin. Invest. 44:1277–1286.

Yalow, R. S., S. M. Glick, J. Roth, and S. Berson. 1964. Radioimmunoassay of human plasma ACTH. J. Clin. Endocrinol. 24:1219–1225.

4

Gonadal
Development

GONADAL DEVELOPMENT

Two normal sex chromosomes are required for the maturation of germ cells (Arey, 1965; Donovan and Van Der Werff Ten Bosch, 1965; and Federman, 1967). Absence of germ cells results in the occurrence of afollicular streak gonads. The absence of one X chromosome (45X) apparently does not affect the intrauterine gonadal structure up to the third month of gestation, but subsequent growth fails to occur. These phenomena are due to the fact that meiotic division, which begins at 2 mo of embryonic life, is impossible in the abnormal germ cell whereas mitotic division is normal. It is probable that two normal chromosones are necessary for crossing over in meiosis I, at which stage there is an exchange of genetic material. A further requirement for follicular development is the ability of oocytes to organize a surrounding granulosa cell layer as they reach the stage of meiosis I. This structure now comprises the primordial follicle which organizes the stroma into a thecal layer. Disturbance of any of these stages renders the ovary incapable of response to stimulation.

A thickening of celomic epithelium by the fourth week of embryonic life is the earliest stage of gonadal development. Primary sex cords grow down from the celomic epithelium into the mesenchymal structure of the gonad. Gonadal development is essentially identical in both sexes up to this point (undifferentiated gonad). Germ cells derived from extragonadal elements in the entoderm of the yolk sac caudal to the embryonic disk migrate to the gonad. These cells are necessary for further gonadal development, and, in their absence, gonadal agenesis occurs. These germ cells at this stage are bipotential, being capable of becoming either sperm cells or ova. The X and Y chromosomes determine their eventual location in the undifferentiated gonad and their subsequent development. By 6 wk of gonadal development the total content of germ cells is approximately 100,000. Testicular differentiation takes place between 6–8 wk of gestation. At this time, there is appearance of medullary primary sex cords or primitive tubules and formation of a limiting membranous tunica and cleft separating deeper layers from surface epithelium. These changes are characteristic of testicular development, and their absence represents the stage of a quiescent primitive ovary. This process of differentiation is dependent on the chromosomal constitution which confers inductor capabilities to the germ cells and on the mesenchymal receptivity. In the presence of the Y chromosome, testicular development proceeds with disappearance of the cortex and persistence of the medullary portion. Primary sex cords form the seminiferous tubules, and the cells of these cords become the Sertoli or sustentacular cells. Mesenchymal cells which surround the tubules become the Leydig or interstitial cells. Testicular descent takes place at the 28th wk of gestation. During this process the testes, gubernaculum, and the epididymis (which is partly derived from the tubules) migrate as a unit into the inguinal canal preceded by a sac of peritoneum, into the scrotum. The process is completed at about the first 4–6 wk of extrauterine life, by which time there is elongation of the vas deferens, disintegration of the gubernaculum, and enlargement of the testes. Wolffian ducts become the vasa deferentia, seminal vesicles, and epididymis, and Müllerian primordia disappear. The prostate is derived from the urethra except for the utricle which is a Müllerian remnant.

In the presence of the XX chromosomal constitution, the process of ovarigenesis takes place. Ovarian formation from the undifferentiated gonad occurs later than testicular differentiation. There is rapid oogonial development at 8–10 wk but it is not until 14 wk of gestation that a number of germ cells are surrounded by precapsular cells derived from the sex cords, while all others not destined to persist undergo degenerative changes. Nuclear maturation takes place at 15–20 wk and most oogonia are transformed into oocytes. The thickened cortex with maturing germ cells is now penetrated by vascular ingrowths perpendicular to the surface and divided into secondary sex cords. Capillaries originating in the mesonephric area separate the cortex from the medulla. The Müllerian primordia grow caudad and meet in the midline, giving rise to the Fallopian tubes, uterus, and upper third of the vagina. Simultaneously, there is regression of the Wolffian system.

Development of external genitalia in both sexes is from a common anlage. In females, the genital tubercle gives rise to the clitoris. With some elongation, this forms the penis in the male. The labia minora in the female are derived from the genital folds, which, in the male, fuse to form the ventral raphe, which displaces the urethral opening to the tip of the penis. The labia majora are formed from the genital swellings, which, in the male, fuse in the midline to form the scrotum.

The final stage in development of the ovaries takes place from 20 wk to time of birth. At this time, there is envelopment of the oocytes with granulosa cells which are associated with capillaries but are not endothelial in origin. These cells enclose the closest oocyte with a single layer of flat cells, with the resulting formation of the primary follicle. By this process eventually all of the germ cells are converted to follicles. Perivascular cells not involved in this process ultimately form the interfollicular stroma. By the time the ovum becomes part of the ovarian follicle, the nucleus has entered phase I of meiosis, at which stage it remains for a variable period until further follicular development is stimulated. This quiescent stage may be quite short, as any oocyte in the primordial follicle may enlarge up to threefold and resume maturation. Associated with this change is maturation of the Graafian follicle with proliferation of a multilayer granulosa, formation of antrum, and a thecal layer with a rich vascular supply. At any step in this maturation process, however, regression may take place, with eventual replacement by connective tissue. It is probable that there is no degeneration of ova in the primary follicle. Most of these changes which occur during fetal life take place at the junction of the cortex and the anatomically minor medulla. It is clear, therefore, that the cycle of formation, ripening, and atresia of follicles is characteristic of fetal ovarian existence. The medullary remnant is made up of cords, nodules, and rete tubules. The medulla persists beyond fetal life as the hilus of the ovary. At birth, the female ovaries contain 400,000–500,000 ova, of which only about 400 will eventually be extruded by ovulation. Variable degrees of atresia is the fate of the rest of the ova.

OVARY FROM BIRTH TO PUBERTY

At birth, each ovary measures 2 cm in diameter, and the bulk of the gland is made up of primordial follicles in a variety of pre-atretic developmental stages. The largest number of primordial follicles exists just prior to birth, after which time there is a rapid decrease. The partial follicular maturation and regression changes seen in fetal life continue into infancy and childhood. After follicular atresia, the cortical stroma accumulates as a connective tissue layer beneath the epithelium, most of these cells being theca residua. Stromal deposition and increase of hilar blood vessels comprise the major growth of the ovary between childhood and puberty.

The prepubertal ovary contains a hilar area with many blood vessels and some medullary remnants with a peripheral cortex of stroma and follicles at various stages of maturity, but without any corpus luteum or evidence of ovulation.

DISORDERS OF SEXUAL DEVELOPMENT

The determinant potencies of the X and Y chromosomes in sexual differentiation and development are described above. It is clear that, in the absence of the Y chromosome, sexual development progresses essentially along female lines. It is now evident that the influence of the Y chromosome and presence of the testes on development of secondary and accessory sexual characteristics are probably dependent on both steroid and nonsteroid secretions from the testes. Early male development, such as that of the Wolffian system, is not dependent on androgens, and it is likely that peptide inductors from the testes may underlie these early stages. The influence of the sex chromosomes may be affected by the numbers and quality of the chromosome structures. Aberrations in the complement of X or Y, therefore, strongly affect development of the sexual characteristics. Several clinical entities are known to result from errors either in disjunction of chromosomes or from other abnormalities.

The normal chromosomal complement in the human species is 22 pairs of autosomes and 2 sex chromosomes, the female containing 2 X chromosomes, *i.e.*, 44 plus XX, whereas the male complement is 44 plus XY. The chromosome karyotype is a systematized distribution of chromosomes from a single cell, the cells being arrested in the metaphase. Chromosomal pairs are arrayed and numbered according to morphologic characteristics, with special emphasis on the relative lengths of the arms (long or short) and the location of the centromere. The X chromosomes are identified on the basis of their resemblance to the larger, medium-sized autosomes with submedian centromeres (groups 6–12). The Y chromosome shows morphologic characteristics of the very short acrocentric autosomes of groups 21–22.

Errors in chromosomal constitution may arise from abnormal replication during gametogenesis or from faulty mitotic division in the zygote after fertilization. Aneuploidy refers to the presence of a different number of chromosomes than is characteristic of the species. This abnormality may be the result of nondisjunction which may occur either during mitotic or meiotic division, and is a failure of separation of a pair of sister chromatids or members of a pair of homologous chromosomes during the anaphase. Loss of a chromosome from one or both of two daughter cells during anaphase lag may also result in aneuploidy.

Other chromosomal structural errors include mosaicism and chimerism. Mosaicism refers to the presence in individuals of two or more cell lines which differ in chromosomal constitution but originate in a single zygote. This type of error occurs only during faulty mitosis after fertilization has occurred. Embryos derived from gametes of abnormal chromosomal characteristics may undergo further errors of replication. It is likely that aging, especially in females, is associated with a gradual and slight increase in aneuploidy. Chimerism refers to the presence of two or more cell lines, each from a different genetic origin. Clinical manifestations are dependent on this admixture of cell lines. The classical example of chimerism is the freemartin, which is a common form of hermaphroditism in cattle in which anastomotic placental channels permit the admixture of hemopoietic and primoidial germ cells between binovular twins of opposite sex. Structural errors in chromosomes may be due to breakage, partial deletion, and improper restitution of broken fragments of the chromosomes. It is likely that an interchange of chromosomal fragments between X and Y during their alignment during meiosis I of spermatogenesis in the father may explain the presence of both testes and ovaries in certain forms of true hermaphroditism, and in rare phenotypic males with the XX karyotype without mosaicism.

The Y chromosome transmits the male-determining characteristics and can induce testicular development even in the presence of two X chromosomes as in Klinefelter's syndrome. The short arm of the Y is apparently most important in determination of masculine development. The trait of hairy ear lobes is also determined by the Y chromosome as an unpaired trait.

The presence of paired X chromosomes is required for differentiation of the bipotential primitive gonad into the ovary. Failure of prenatal ovarian development occurs in patients with the XO chromosomal complement (45XO). Apparently the long and short arms are involved in ovarian development.

The presence of a stainable chromatin mass at the periphery of the nucleus in over 24% of cells with well-preserved nuclei is characteristic of the female. This phenomenon is dependent on the fact that the X chromosome which gives rise to the sex chromatin completes its DNA synthesis later than any other chromosome in the cell, hence, the staining property which is due to DNA. The size of the nuclear chromatin mass is related to the constitution of the X chromosomes, so that a small amount is seen in patients with partly deleted chromosome material, as is XX^D, and a large amount is seen in the presence of increase chromosome material as with the X isochrome, as is XX^I.

Table 4.1 summarizes the various factors involved in sexual differentiation as well as development of secondary characteristics. Examples of chromosomal abnormalities and clinical disorders due to nondisjunction of sex chromosomes during meiotic division in the parental germ cells are shown in table 4.2. A classification of anomalous sexual differentiation with the significant clinical features is presented in table 4.3.

THE MENSTRUAL CYCLE

The human menstrual cycle refers to a pattern of events which include Graafian follicle development and maturation, proliferative changes in the endometrium, ovulation, corpus luteum development with associated secretory changes in the endometrium, and culminating in menstruation, the sloughing of decidual layers of the endometrium. While the overt changes are seen in the ovaries and the endometrium, systemic manifestations reflecting

Table 4.1. Factors in Sexual Differentiation and Development

Characteristic	Origin	Mechanism of differentiation	Identifying features
Chromosomal sex	Sex chromosomes of parental germ cells	Normal: chromosomal composition of sperm Abnormal: nondisjunction during meiosis in parental germ cells Nondisjunction or lag in early mitotic divisions Chromosomal breakage	Karyotype analysis
X-chromatin	Heterochromatic X chromosomes	Partial inactivation and heterochromatization of all chromosomes in excess of one	Buccal, neutrophil or other somatic cells
Y-body	Y chromosome	Distal segment of long arm of Y	Buccal, neutrophil or other somatic cells
Gonadal sex	Ovaries	Presence of genes on two X chromosones	Histologic appearance
	Testes	Presence of genes on Y chromosomes	Histologic appearance
Genital ducts	Müllerian or Wolffian ducts	Intrinsic tendency to feminize in absence of androgens which stimulate Wolffian system	Morphologic appearance
External genitalia	Genital tubercle, urethral and labioscrotal folds, urogenital sinus	As above; masculinization requires androgen stimulation before 12th week	Examination; urethroscopy; X-ray contrast study

Secondary sexual characteristics	Hypothalamic and suprahypo-thalamic centers; pituitary FSH, LH, ovaries, testes, adrenals	Suprahypothalamic and hypothalamic centers: gonadotropin-releasing hormones Gonads: responsiveness to FSH and LH Target organs: responsiveness depends on presence of cytosol receptor	Abnormalities: virilized female: adrenal hyperplasia or maternal androgens; incompletely differentiated male: insufficient androgen from fetal testes, or end-organ refractoriness such as due to absence of cytosol receptor

Overt secondary sexual characteristics (female): breast development, rounded contours, growth of reproductive tract, ovulation, menstruation (all due to gonadal hormone release under tonic and cyclic control)

Overt secondary sexual characteristics (male): sexual hair pattern, voice, muscular development, phallic size (secondary to release of androgens under tonic control)

Table 4.2. Chromosomal Abnormalities Due to Nondisjunction during Meiosis

Abnormality	Oocyte	Meiosis (ovum + polar body)	Product of Conception[a]	Meiosis (2 sperm)	Spermatocyte
None	44 XX	22 X + 22 X	44 XX or 44 XY	22 X + 22 Y	44 XY
Maternal nondisjunction	44 XX	22 X (p.b.[b]) 22 XX	44 XXX	22 Y 22 X	44 XY
	44 XX	22 O (p.b.) 22 O	44 XXY 44 XO	22 Y 22 X	44 XY
Paternal nondisjunction	44 XX	22 XX (p.b.) 22 X +	44 YO 44 XXY	22 Y 22 XY	44 XY
	44 XX	22 X (p.b.)	44 XO	22 O	44 XY

[a]Products of conception: 44 XX, normal female; 44 XY, normal male; 44 XXX, superfemale; 44 XXY, Klinefelter's syndrome; 44 XO, gonadal dysgenesis (Turner's); 44 YO, incompatible with life.
[b]p.b., polar body.

Table 4.3. Anomalous Sexual Differentiation in the Female

Disorders	Clinical features
Gonadal differentiation: Gonadal dysgenesis, true hermaphroditism	Attributable to anomalous sex chromosomes, ranging from XO, XX, XX^D and variants or mosaicism; genital duct and external sexual characteristics as well as hormonal sex consistent with gonadal histology; frequently associated with mental retardation and physical abnormalities
Female pseudohermaphroditism Congenital virilizing adreno-cortical hyperplasia; exposure to excess maternal androgens; other factors	Positive sex chromatin XX karyotype; gonads and internal ducts female in type; external genitalia may range from clitoromegaly to simulant cryptorchid male
Unclassified Absence or anomalous development of uterus and Fallopian tubes; vaginal agenesis; postpubertal virilism and infertility	Sex chromosomes normal; ambiguous genitalia not a prominent feature

the effects of the gonadal hormones also take place. These include changes in breast size, vaginal secretions, emotional state, and other biologic functions. The control of these cyclic changes is mediated by the hypothalamic-pituitary axis as well as by suprahypothalamic and infrahypophysial factors which influence this regulation.

The time of onset of menstrual cyclicity, menarche, is usually at the age of 13 yr in the United States, but this landmark is influenced by climatic, ethnic, and familial factors. At birth, the female individual possesses a fund of several hundred thousands of potential ova, but cyclic release of ova does not start until the age of menarche. The reason for the latent period is not clear, but there are several factors which deserve consideration. These include the sensitivity of the hypothalamic nuclei to negative or positive feedback control by ambient levels of gonadal hormones and to suprahypothalamic and central nervous system influences. In addition, the responsiveness of the ovarian Graafian follicle cells to gonadotropic hormones has been shown to be age- and, perhaps, body development-related. Some consideration of the maturation of the hypothalamic-pituitary and ovarian axis was presented in the preceding chapter.

The Adult Ovary and the Menstrual Cycle

The principal functional unit of the adult ovary is the follicle, consisting of an ovum and two layers of tissue, an inner band of granulosa cells and an outer vascularized mantle, the thecal cells. The follicles present in the ovary show varying degrees of maturity reflected by the amount of granulosa proliferation, appearance and degree of thecal layer thickening, and antral size. Only a few follicles reach maturity since most regress by atresia.

Stages of Follicular Growth

In the first stage of follicular growth, the oocyte enlarges and the single originally flat granulosa layer becomes cuboidal and proliferates into a multilayer band of tissue. This layer receives its nutrition from the thecal layer since it lacks an intrinsic vascularity. The proliferation of granulosa cells results in formation of a multilayer granulosa layer with some intercellular spaces. This is surrounded by a more concentrated thecal layer (figs. 4.1 and 4.2). As oocyte growth and enlargement continue, there is a widening of the granulosa layer where fluid-filled intercellular spaces appear secondary to either cellular liquefaction or to secretion. These later coalesce to form the antrum. The liquor folliculi then becomes a transudate of blood filtered through the granulosa layer. The follicular antrum is not in contact with the ovum, which is encased in a random mound of granulosa cells, the cumulus oophorus. As the antrum enlarges, the cells of the cumulus enlarge and the

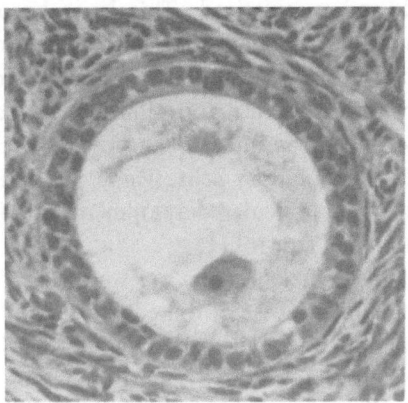

Figure 4.1. Follicular development; a maturing follicle at intermediate stage. The oocyte is surrounded by a single layer of granulosa cells. (Photograph courtesy of L. E. Watkins, M.D.)

granulosa cells are compressed (fig. 4.2). Vascular canals from the theca traverse the granulosa layer to supply the ovum, forming the corona radiata. The ovum is now encased in a zona pellucida, which is made up of a polysaccharide fluid produced by the granulosa.

Formation of the theca occurs at the time of antrum formation. The thecal cells are arranged concentrically in a sheath around the follicle, and consist of an inner layer, the theca interna, in which the cells enlarge rapidly,

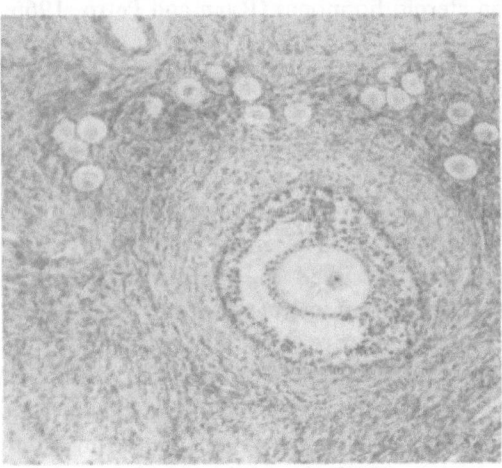

Figure 4.2. Several developmental stages in follicular growth are seen in this panoramic view. In the mature Graafian follicle, the oocyte is seen encased in a zona pellucida. Liquor folliculi fills the follicular cavity. The ovum is encased in a zona pellucida. (Photograph courtesy of L. E. Watkins, M.D.)

become vacuolated, and vascularized. This layer becomes lipid-laden, presumably for nutrition of the granulosa cells. The theca externa is made up of compressed connective tissue without muscle or elastic tissue components. Follicle growth now proceeds to maturation, with expansion of the antrum and enlargement of the theca interna. The ovum eventually becomes supported on a hillock of granulosa cells. There is no further growth of the oocyte at this time, and follicular development and function come under gonadotropic direction and control.

Development of the follicle may be arrested at any stage, and regression and atresia follow. In this process of follicular atresia, there is disruption and disappearance of the granulosa cells and they become flattened and resemble connective tissue. Obliteration of the antrum leaves a ribbon-like streak surrounded by markedly reduced theca. The oocyte degenerates *in situ.* These atretic follicles may persist for considerable periods before complete disappearance. Occasionally, cyst formation in the atretic follicles may occur, the process involving a distension of the cavity with fluid. These cysts may be found in normal ovaries during the reproductive years. There is increased follicular atresia during pregnancy. In chronic inflammatory disease, the appearance of numerous follicular cysts may cause cystic ovary disease. The corpus fibrosum is formed from degeneration and fibrosis of the follicular cyst.

Steroidogenesis in the Ovaries

Several elements in ovarian tissue are capable of, and participate in biosynthesis of, the ovarian steroid hormones (Ryan and Petro, 1966; Mikhail, 1970). Several of the steps in the biosynthetic pathway are identical to those in the adrenal cortex, and, in males, in the testes. The eventual substrate for hormone synthesis is acetyl CoA, which is utilized in the synthesis of cholesterol. Cholesterol is converted to the intermediate pregnenolone (Δ^5 pregnen, 3β-ol, 20-one) and isocaproic acid by the desmolase system. This enzyme is activated by cAMP, which is released by membrane adenyl cyclase, which is stimulated by LH. The membrane receptor specificity for the peptide hormones was described in Chapter 1. Figure 4.3 presents the pathways of the synthesis of estrogens from pregnenlone in the ovaries. Pregnenolone has two alternative fates. One synthetic pathway is dependent on the presence of the enzyme 17α-hydroxylase, which converts pregnenolone to 17α-hydroxypregnenolone. A desmolase enzyme then cleaves off the side chain from 17α-hydroxypregnenolone, resulting in the formation of dehydroepiandrosterone (DHEA). DHEA is biologically active as a weak androgen. This series of reactions is mediated by microsomal enzymes and is called the Δ^5 pathway. DHEA is converted to androstenedione by the HSD system which consists of two reactions, a 3β-dehydrogenase and a Δ^5 iso-

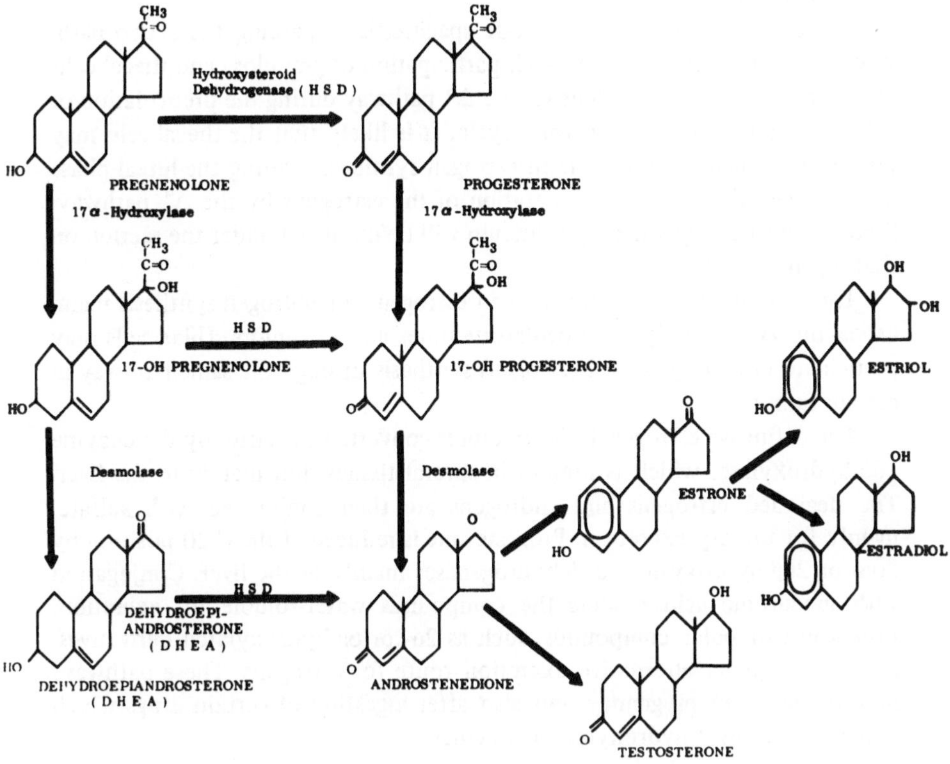

Figure 4.3. Steroidogenesis in the ovary. Two pathways are depicted—the Δ^5 pathway is predominant during the folliculoid phase, whereas the Δ^4 pathway, which provides both progesterone and estrogens, is active in the luteal phase of the cycle.

merase. Androstenedione has two alternative fates, namely reduction by a 17β-dehydrogenase to testosterone, which is a powerful androgen, or to a 19-hydroxylated derivative of androstenedione. The 19-hydroxylation step is followed successively by 19-aldo and 19-carboxylic acid formation, which are converted to estrone by oxidation at carbons 1 and 2. Estrone is then reduced at the ketone group at C 17 to form 17β-estradiol, which is the definitive estrogen. The alternative fate of pregnenolone involves the conversion to progesterone by the HSD enzyme system. Progesterone is then hydroxylated at C 17 by the microsomal 17α-hydroxylase. Cleavage of the side chain of 17α-hydroxyprogesterone is catalyzed by the desmolase enzyme system, with the resultant formation of androstenedione. This series of microsomal reactions, transforming pregnenolone eventually to androstenedione, is termed the Δ^4 pathway.

There are relative cell and phase specificities regarding these two pathways. There is a synergistic two-cell participation of granulosa and thecal cells in the production of estrogens via the Δ^5 pathway during the preovulation or folliculoid phase of the menstrual cycle. It is likely that the thecal cells may utilize preformed progesterone in estrogen synthesis. During the luteal phase of the cycle, there is active generation of the estrogens by the Δ^4 pathway. Steroid synthesis by the corpus luteum will be discussed under the section on that organ.

The ovarian stroma participates in estrogen and androgen synthesis mainly via the Δ^5 pathway in anovulatory states and in tumors. Hilar cells may participate in androgen (and estrogen) synthesis through the same pathway in certain tumors.

The definitive estrogen 17β-estradiol is converted to estriol by the enzyme 16α-hydroxylase, which is present in several tissues, but mainly in the liver. The degraded estrogens and androgens are then conjugated with sulfate, mainly for urinary excretion. Progesterone is reduced at the C 20 position by 20α- or 20β-hydroxysteroid dehydrogenases mainly in the liver. Conjugation with glucuronic acid renders the compounds water-soluble for excretion. Formation of polar compounds, such as 2α- or 6β-hydroxylated derivatives, may represent an alternative excretion route for estrogens. These pathways may be active in pregnancy and also after ingestion of certain drugs which induce microsomal hydroxylation enzymes.

Ovulation

The final maturation step of the developing follicle consists of rupture of the distended follicle and extrusion of the ovum. With fluid engorgement of the antrum, the cumulus attachment to the rest of the granulosa layer is pinched and atrophied. The antral engorgement distorts the capsule of the ovary, but apparently pressure *per se* is not responsible for the process of ovulation. Orientation of the follicle toward the surface is determined by formation of a wedgelike cone of thecal tissue. When the thecal cone (stigma) is just beneath the superficial epithelium, avascular necrosis of the superficial capsule occurs. Ovulation takes place from the stigma. The process involves the dissolution of mucopolysaccharide cement in the capsule. This process is activated by LH.

Corpus Luteum

The formation of the corpus luteum is a direct consequence of final maturation of the follicle and the process of ovulation. After discharge of the ovum, there is a collapse of the follicle with the appearance of a crumbled pattern which is very characteristic and is regarded as a reliable indication that ovulation has taken place. The corpus luteum has an inherent life span of 14–16 days unless it is restimulated by chorionic gonadotropin from the trophoblast. The life cycle of the corpus luteum consists of three progressive stages prior to retrogression. The proliferative stage occurs immediately following follicular rupture. The granulosa layer of the follicle becomes transformed into large, vacuolated, and lipid-laden cells, as the lutein cells. This zone is surrounded by a perigranulosal vascular wreath. The stage of vascularization is characterized by an invasion of the layer of lutein cells by blood vessels from the theca. Limited amounts of hemorrhage into the luminal edge may occur, but on occasion the cavity may become distended with blood. The theca interna virtually disappears after undergoing retrogressive changes. At this stage the corpus luteum appears as a hemorrhagic-looking structure of 10–12 mm in diameter, often forming a slight mound on the surface of the ovary. The stage of maturity correlates with the phase of progesterone effect on the endometrium. The lutein zone assumes a yellowish color due to the presence of carotene in the lipid. The lutein layer is divided into folds and alveoli by septa pushed downward from the theca. Some of the cells of the thecal layer may themselves show evidence of luteinization as theca lutein or paralutein cells which are distinguished from granulosa lutein cells by being smaller. Along the luminal edge of the lutein cells, a zone of fibroblastic tissue forms, separating the lutein layer from the cavity which now contains unresorbed elements of the previous hemorrhage. At this stage, the corpus luteum may range from 10–20 mm in diameter and may be seen through the surface of the ovary. Maximum growth of the corpus luteum occurs about 4–6 days before menstrual bleeding. The stage of retrogression of the corpus luteum is characterized by fatty degeneration, fibrosis, and hyalinization of the lutein zone, with the elements in the cavity showing cicatrization. The yellow color may disappear after weeks to months with the eventual appearance of the corpus albicans which slowly decreases in size.

Steroidogenesis in the Corpus Luteum

During the luteal phase of the menstrual cycle, steroid synthesis proceeds through the Δ^4 pathway described above (Ryan and Petro, 1966; Mikhail, 1970). In this manner, appropriate amounts of both estrogens and progesterone are produced for continued preparation of the endometrium for implantation of a fertilized ovum. Both hormones suppress the release of pituitary LH. This results in degeneration of the corpus luteum, which has an inherent life span of 14–16 days unless further stimulated (see later in this chapter).

Hormonal Events in the Menstrual Cycle

The earliest stages of follicular development are independent of gonadotropic control (Abraham et al, 1972; Ross et al, 1970). The inability of the undifferentiated theca to secrete adequate amounts of estrogen is probably responsible for a lack of ovarian response early in the cycle (Goldenberg, Reiter, and Ross, 1973). Proliferation of granulosa cells is stimulated only after the theca interna becomes responsive to gonadotropins and secretes estrogens. FSH initiates development of several follicular units, but in each cycle, only one reaches maturity, in which stage it is responsive to the LH surge which induces ovulation. Plasma levels of FSH show an early rise in the first few days of the follicular phase. This is followed by a decline in the second part of the follicular phase, reaching lowest levels late in this phase. An abrupt rise in FSH then occurs just prior to ovulation, followed by a nadir 10 days later in the luteal phase. A slight rise occurs around the time of onset of menstrual bleeding, probably representing the beginning of the early FSH rise of the folliculoid phase of the subsequent cycle.

Plasma LH levels begin to increase in the second part of the folliculoid phase. This is followed by a sharp rise to about 5 times the basal level, followed by a fall to basal levels, with a further drop during the luteal phase (fig. 4.4). Detailed studies revealed that there is an episodic pattern in LH levels probably related to the sleep cycle; this pattern is also seen during the LH surge. The levels of plasma estradiol fluctuate in relation to those of the gonadotropins. During menstruation, the levels of estradiol are quite low. There is a gradual rise during the early follicular phase followed by a sharp increase during the late follicular phase. A peak level is reached about 12–24 hr before the LH peak; this is followed by a drop at the time of ovulation. During the luteal phase, there is again a rise in estradiol, followed by a decrease during menstrual bleeding.

The midcycle surge of pituitary gonadotropins results from the rapid increase in estradiol. Urinary studies reveal similar rises of estrone and estriol. This effect of estrogens on the surge of FSH and LH is dependent on certain temporal relationships (Cargille et al., 1973). Estradiol administration sufficient to cause an estrogen rise in the midfollicular phase of the menstrual cycle is also capable of inducing a rise in LH and FSH within 12–24 hr. Administration of estradiol at an earlier time in the follicular phase (days 3–5) is followed by a dissociation in the responses of the gonadotropins, with occurence of an LH surge but without a similar rise in FSH. Immediate

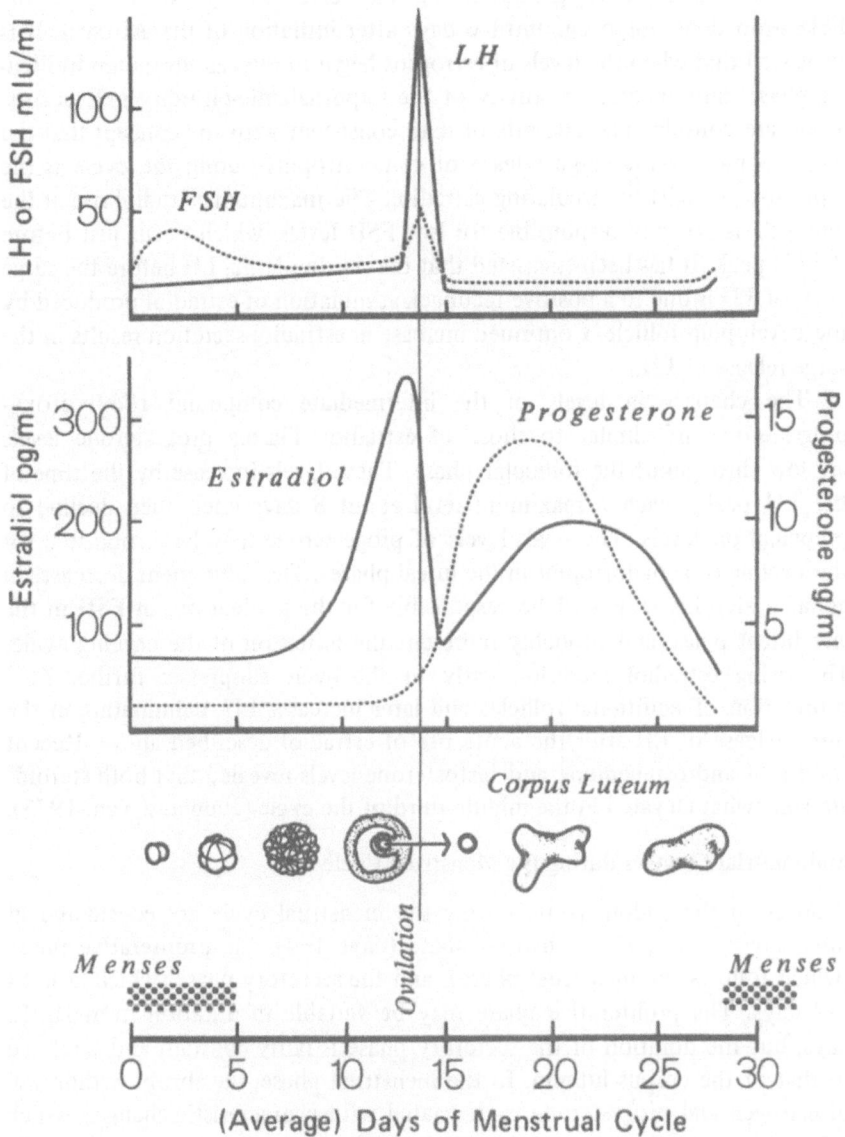

Figure 4.4. The events of the menstrual cycle. Cyclic changes in the levels of FSH, LH, estradiol, and progesterone, as well as in the morphology of the follicle, are depicted. The endometrial changes during the phases are described in the text. The operation of a negative-feedback circuit, as well as an example of a positive-feedback circuit involving estradiol and the secretion of FSH and LH, are described in the text. (Reprinted by permission of A. L. Nichols, M.D.)

suppression of serum FSH occurs if exogenous estradiol is started on the day of menses; but if the exogenous estrogen is started on day 9 of the cycle, the FSH drop does not occur until 6 days after initiation of the estrogen. It is suggested that when the levels of estrogens begin to increase in the midfollicular phase, an increased sensitivity of the hypothalamic-pituitary axis occurs. There are considerable amounts of data consistent with the concept that the major signal for the surge release of gonadotropins during the cycle is the rapid rise (or fall) of circulating estradiol. The maximum estradiol rise at the midcycle is possibly responsible for low FSH levels, which occur just before the LH peak. It has been suggested that the rise in plasma LH before the surge peak of LH is due to a positive feedback stimulation of estradiol produced by the developing follicle. Continued increase in estradiol secretion results in the surge release of LH.

The changes in levels of the intermediate compound 17α-hydroxy-progesterone are similar to those of estradiol. Plasma progesterone levels are low throughout the follicular phase. These levels increase by the time of the LH peak, reach a maximum level about 8 days later, then decline to preovulation levels. The peak levels of progesterone may be responsible for the decline of gonadotropins in the luteal phases. The subsequent decreases in gonadal steroids may well be responsible for the gradual rise in FSH in the late luteal phase and probably represent the initiation of the ensuing cycle. The rising estradiol secretion early in the cycle suppresses further FSH stimulation of additional follicles and later increases LH, culminating in the surge release of LH after the acute rise of estradiol described above. Recent studies of androstenedione and testosterone levels revealed that both steroids are somewhat elevated in the middle third of the cycle (Judd and Yen, 1973).

Endometrial Changes during the Menstrual Cycle

Changes in the endometrium during the menstrual cycle are considered in three phases, viz., the menstrual phase (days 1–4), the proliferative phase (which follows the menstrual phase), and the secretory phase (which lasts 14 ± 2 days. The proliferative phase may be variable in duration from 10–12 days, but the duration of the secretory phase is fairly constant and is related to that of the corpus luteum. In the menstrual phase, the abrupt withdrawal of estrogen and progesterone is associated with characteristic changes, which culminate in the sloughing of the decidual cells.Endometrial tissue, previously supported for sufficient periods and with sufficient amounts of estrogen and progesterone, on losing this support, abruptly undergoes certain morphologic alterations. The predeciduum is first deprived of nutriment, there is shrinkage of the decidual cells, autolysis, and the layer becomes thinner. The stromal support of the superficial capillaries undergoes autolysis, the caliber of the spiral vessels decreases, and constriction of the vessels results in local ischemia. Further stromal shrinkage is followed by kinking of the coiled arteries. Constriction of these spiral vessels at the basal parts closest to the myometrium occurs. Subsequent vasodilation in these vessels is followed by bleeding and sloughing of the endometrium. This process lasts for approximately 4 days during which fibrinolysins released from this tissue aid in lysis of clots. There are recent data which suggest that decreased lysosomal integrity is probably the basis of the destruction of the decidual cells and the sloughing.

In the proliferative phase of the menstrual cycle, there is cessation of menstrual bleeding and endometrial desquamation. Increasing estrogen levels induce rapid re-epithelialization and the vascularity is restored. The early proliferative phase (days 4–7) is characterized by the presence of glands which are short and narrow, with considerable mitotic activity. The surface epithelium showing regenerative changes, and the stroma showing few mitoses, are compact with stellate- or spindle-shaped cells with large nuclei and scanty cytoplasm. In the middle proliferative phase (days 7–10), there is the beginning of pseudostratification of nuclei with the glands appearing longer and somewhat curved. The stroma shows some edematous changes, and there is significant mitotic activity. The scanty cytoplasm and stromal edema produce the naked nucleus effect. At this stage, also, the surface epithelium is covered with columnar epithelium. In the late proliferative phase, the actively growing glands show numerous mitoses and pseudostratification of the nuclei, and appear tortuous. The stroma shows active growth with numerous mitoses.

The secretory phase of the menstrual cycle lasts about 14 days, the first half confined largely to changes in the glandular epithelium, and the latter half confined mainly to changes in the stroma. Stromal changes provide a method of dating the stages of the phase. Basal vacuolation is the earliest morphologic indication that ovulation has occurred; this is first noted on about day 16 in most glands, associated with little or no mitotic activity in the glands or in the stoma. By day 17, there is a characteristic accumulation of glycogen in subnuclear vacuoles, with the cytoplasm located above the nuclei of the glands. Little mitotic activity is noted in the stroma or glands at this time. Discharge of glycogen into the cytoplasm is noted by day 18, at which time the nuclei move toward the bases of the cells. The characteristic lining up of the nuclei above the vacuoles is best seen on day 17, and this serves as an excellent indication of recent ovulation. Secretory activity of the glands is evident by days 18–22, with appearance of loose feathery material in the lumina, providing the best milieu for implantation at around days 20 – 22.

Stromal edema is most striking around days 22 and 23, at which time the stromal cells show dark dense nuclei with filamentous cytoplasm. This morphologic alteration probably facilitates implantation by decreasing tissue resistance. A periarterial predecidual reaction noted by days 23 and 24 is regarded as a protective mechanism against premature vascular disruption and as a supportive framework for neovascularization. Involutional changes in the endometrium evident by day 24 consist of marked periarteriolar predicidual collections, active mitoses, and a decrease of stromal edema. Within the next 2 days, there is lymphocytic infiltration of the stroma and edema in the perioarteriolar areas; this is followed by polymorphonuclear infiltration throughout the stroma and an increase in the predecidua. Focal areas of necrosis and stromal hemorrhage associated with exhaustion of the glands are seen by day 28.

Systemic Changes during the Menstrual Cycle

Several systemic changes are noted during the menstrual cycle; these vary in degree depending on the organ systems involved and individual sensitivities to these changes. Several neurologic manifestations may be associated with phases of menstrual cycle. For example, migraine headaches are often related to ovulatory cycles and may be relieved by pregnancy and anovulatory periods. This phenomenon is probably not related to alteration in water or electrolyte balance. Nevertheless, it is likely that these episodes may be related to relative amounts of estrogen and progresterone in the circulation. Ovulatory suppression by progestins may alleviate attacks of migraine, whereas estrogen-progestin combinations may not. Increased cerebral cortical activity is noted during menses, and may result in increased seizure activity in susceptible individuals. Despite suggestions that altered sodium and water balance may be related to this phenomenon, recent data are more consistent with the concept that the increased cortical activity is noted during menses and may result in increased seizure activity in susceptible individuals. Psychologic changes during the cycle are often noted in the premenstrual phase when there may be increased libido, irritability, depression, aggression, and violent behavior in certain hyperactive women.

In the premenstrual period, lowered estrogen and increased skin sebum may be associated with aggravation of acne vulgaris. Many other cutaneous manifestations may occur or be exacerbated in the premenstrual period, including aphthous stomatitis, pyorrhea, Vincent's angina, and chronic ulcerative colitis. Perhaps variations in the release of β-MSH are responsible for some increased pigmentation around the eyes, areolae, and perioral area about 1 wk prior to menstrual bleeding. During the luteal phase of the cycle, increased capillary fragility and decreased platelets may occur in normal individuals. Such tendency is exacerbated in patients with thrombocytopenia purpura, leukemia, and other hematologic disorders. There is a slightly decreased hematocrit and increased blood volume at the end of menstruation in normal women. Menstruation may also affect certain clinical disorders. Attacks of acute intermittent porphyria may be increased during the period of menstrual flow and may be precipitated by exogenous progestins. This is probably ascribable to the effect of this group of steroids on the enzyme δ-aminolevulinic (δ-ALA) synthetase (Perlroth, Marver, and Tschudy, 1965). There are reports which indicate that appendicitis attacks rarely occur during menses. Epistaxis, hyperemia of the turbinates, rhinorrhea, sinus congestion, and asthma attacks have been noted to be precipitated or exacerbated by menstruation.

Alterations in several of the parameters affected by other endocrine glands are also noted during menstruation. The secretion of aldosterone, as well as serum sodium:potassium and the urine sodium:potassium ratios, are affected by the phases of the menstrual cycle. During the follicular phase, the mean value of plasma aldosterone secretion is 140 ng/100 ml, whereas it is increased to 233 ng/100 ml during the luteal phase (Gray et al., 1968). This menstrual cyclicity in aldosterone secretion is obliterated when the cycle is suppressed with an estrogen-progestin combination. The severity of diabetes mellitus and the tendency to acidosis is increased during menstruation. This has been ascribed to a decrease in estrogen levels.

CORPUS LUTEUM OF PREGNANCY

Should fertilization of the ovum take place, the zygote traverses the oviduct toward the endometrium. The progress through the oviduct is hastened by high estrogen levels, and this effect of estrogens is being used clinically for pregnancy control. The site of implantation of the zygote, now at least at morula stage, on the endometrium is usually an area protected from physical trauma. Implantation takes place within 4–6 days after fertilization. Blastocyst formation is followed by the start of production of human chorionic gonadotropin (HCG), a glycoprotein hormone. This hormone is detectable as early as 9 days after implantation and reaches peak levels at 60–80 days of gestation, after which the HCG levels drop to considerably lower levels. The initial persistence and steroidogenesis in the corpus luteum are undoubtedly dependent on the production of HCG. Steroidogenesis in the corpus luteum reaches its peak at 3–4 wk after fertilization and decreases thereafter despite continuing elevation of HCG. Estrogens and progesterone produced by the corpus luteum of pregnancy at this stage inhibit cyclic secretion of pituitary gonadotropins and prevent further ovulation. The various pregnancy tests are based on the levels of HCG in plasma and urine (Mishell et al., 1973).

Despite evidence of maximal development of the corpus luteum of pregnancy by 10–12 wk, it is known that steroid production by the placenta occurs much earlier. Corpus luteum function may continue for several weeks, but may not be essential for continuation of the pregnancy beyond the second missed period. Of 51 pregnant women in whom the corpus luteum was removed before this time, only 17 aborted the fetus (Ask-Upmark,

1926). Previous conclusions that the sole function of HCG is prolongation of corpus luteum life-span may not be valid, as relatively recent data strongly suggest a role of HCG in the function of the fetal zone of the adrenal.

Steroidogenesis in the placenta starts relatively early in pregnancy, and, by 36 days, progesterone is produced in sufficient amounts to maintain a pregnancy in the absence of the corpus luteum. Progesterone serves to maintain the function of the quiescent uterus, and plasma levels of progesterone or urinary levels of pregnanediol in the third trimester serve as indices of placental function. Estrogen production by the placenta reaches significant amounts by the tenth week after the last missed period. The bulk of this elevation is reflected by the levels of estriol sulfate, but estrone and estradiol are also significantly elevated. Considerable data indicate the close relationship between fetal health and urinary estriol excretion. The fetal zone of the adrenal cortex is intimately involved in the production of estrogens in pregnancy. Several enzymatic steps in the formation of estriol sulfate are confined to fetal compartment, and, accordingly, the plasma or urinary levels of estrogens are sensitive indicators of fetal health after the first trimester. Estrogen levels in the amniotic fluid, as well as quantitation of the levels of 16α-hydroxydehydroepiandrosterone, reflect fetal steroidogenesis (Mitchell and Shackleton, 1966).

After 90 days of gestation, the HCG levels drop and plateau at a lower level. Simultaneously, the cells of the fetoplacental unit are fully capable of producing the steroid hormones necessary for the pregnancy. The placenta also produces the following peptide hormones (see fig. 4.5). (1) Chorionic somatomammotropin (HCS) was previously termed placental lactogen (HPL), and is secreted by the syncytiotrophoblast cels until the end of pregnancy. This hormone has several similarities to HGH (growth hormone) in structure, as well as in biologic activity. The production rate is estimated to be over 1 g daily, over 99% of which is in the maternal compartment where it induces lipolysis and provides free fatty acids for maternal metabolism, sparing carbohydrate and protein for fetal metabolism. This action probably contributes to the fasting metabolism state in pregnancy (see the section on diabetic pregnancy in Chapter 11). (2) Production of a placental thyrotropin has been reported, and it has been shown to have biologic activity.

STEROIDOGENESIS IN THE FETOPLACENTAL UNIT

Close metabolic relationship between the maternal and fetal compartments is exemplified by the interplay of steroidogenic tissues during gestation (fig. 4.6) (Villee, 1972). The syncytiotrophoblast is active in the production of estrogen and progesterone, but there are now data to show that the placenta is an incomplete steroidogenic tissue. The steroidogenic cells of the fetus, the

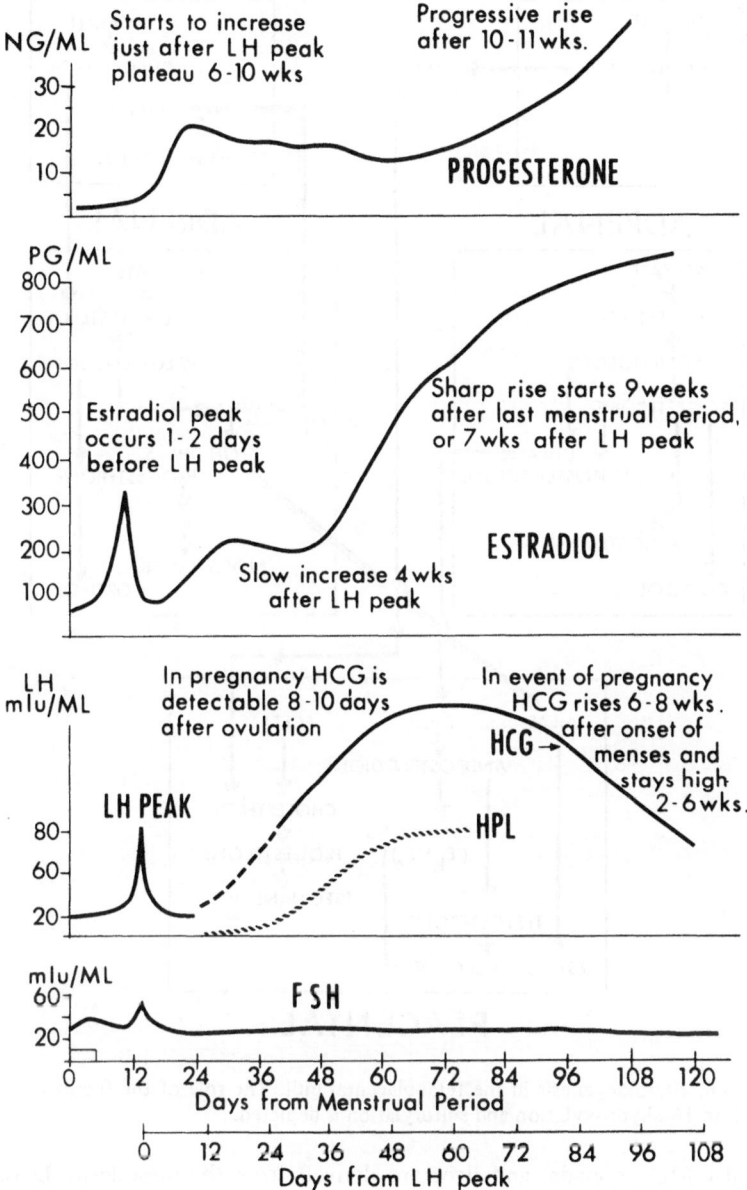

Figure 4.5. Hormonal changes in pregnancy. Maternal plasma or urinary levels of gonadotropic hormones, estrogens, progesterone, and somatomammotropin are depicted.

MATERNAL
liver

FETAL
liver

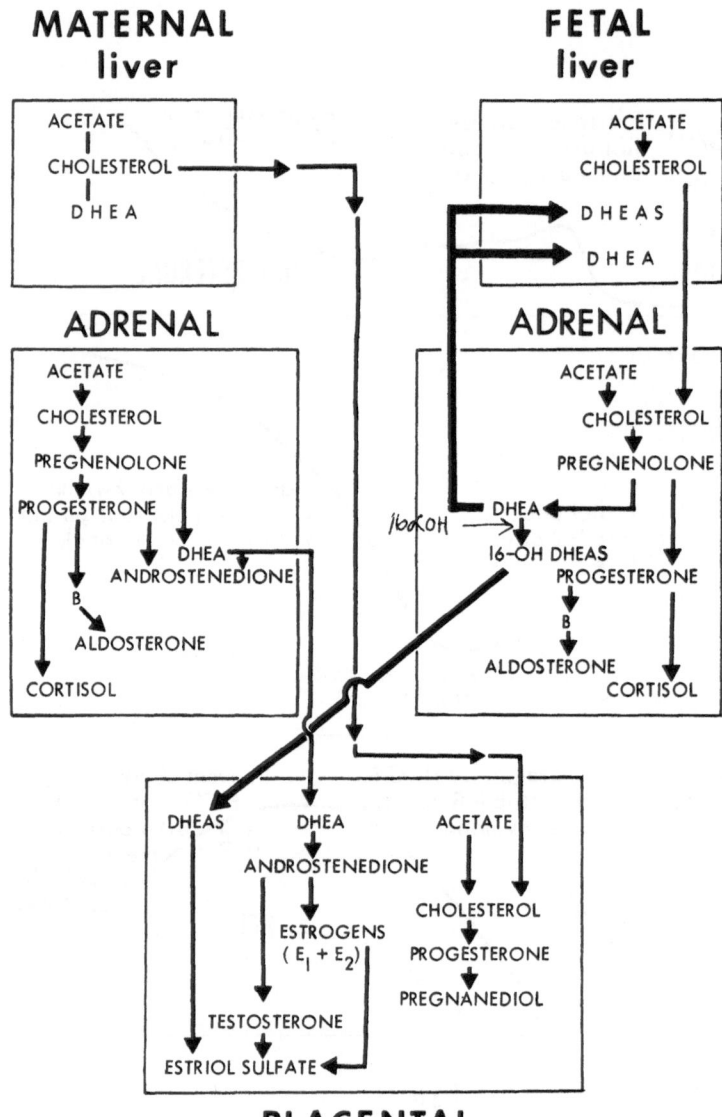

Figure 4.6. Steroidogenesis in the fetal-placental unit. The role of the fetal zone of the adrenals in 16α-hydroxylation and sulfurylation is depicted.

adrenal cortex, gonads, and liver are derived from the mesoderm. Development of the adrenal cortex in the fetus shows that there are probably two relatively discrete areas of the gland, both from morphologic and biosynthetic aspects.

By 5–6 wk of gestation, the adrenal is made up of relatively undifferentiated cells, loosely connected to each other and surrounded by a thin fibrous capsule. By 6–7 wk, the gland divides into a thin outer zone and a wide inner (fetal) zone. Cell maturation proceeds differently in these two areas. The fetal (inner) zone cells show maturation changes without any evidence of mitosis. The outer zone is actively mitotic, and new cells are formed with evidence of slow maturation. There is reason to conclude that the outer zone eventually evolves into the adult adrenal cortex, whereas the inner wide fetal zone, which developed earlier, eventually disappears after having functioned during gestation and in early neonatal life. The fetal zone is known to completely involute by 6 mo after birth.

There is good evidence that cholesterol from the maternal compartment is the precursor for steroidogenesis in the placenta. The fetal compartment is capable of significant conversion of acetate to cholesterol, with activities greatest in the liver, adrenal tissue, and gonadal tissue, in that order. However, it is likely that precursors for steroidogenesis beyond cholesterol may reach the fetus from the maternal or placental compartment.

There are significant differences between the biosynthetic potentials of the placenta and the fetus (table 4.4). Those data make it clear why pregnanediol is a reflection of placental activity, whereas the formation of estriol sulfate is largely dependent on the activity of the fetal adrenal and liver. The fetal zone of the adrenal function is the major site of steroid synthesis in early gestation. Structural maturation in this gland occurs by 6–7 wk of gestation, and increased estrogens are detectable at 15–16 wk. By this time, the adult zone of the adrenal cortex has not yet differentiated structurally. The fetal zone is geared for the Δ^5 pathway, and for sulfurylation of these steroids. These compounds constitute the major steroids in fetal and neonatal

Table 4.4. Steroidogenic Enzymes in Placenta and Fetal Adrenal

Enzyme system	Reaction	Placenta	Fetal adrenal
Hydroxysteroid dehydrogenase	Converts Δ^5, 3β-ol to Δ^4, 3-ketone	Active	Minimal to absent
17 α-hydroxylase	Hydroxylation at C 17 permitting cleavage by 17:20 desmolase	Minimal	Active
17:20 desmolase	Cleavage of side chain of C 21 steroids → KS	Active	Active
Sulfokinase	Sulfurylation of steroids at C 3, *e.g.*, DHEA, DHEAS	Absent	Active
16 α-hydroxylase	Hydroxylation at C 16, *e.g.*, estradiol, estriol	Absent	Active in fetal liver and adrenals
Steroid sulfatase	Removal of sulfate at C 3	Present	Absent

body fluids until the fetal zone involutes (by 6 mo of age) and the adult zone takes over. (Lauritzen, Shackleton, and Mitchell, 1968).

The fetal adrenal uses placentally produced progesterone for further steroid synthesis, *e.g.*, (1) formation of corticosterone via 21-hydroxylase and 11β-hydroxylase reactions; (2) formation of cortisol via 17α-hydroxylase, 21-hydroxylase, and 11β-hydroxylase reactions. The cortisol:corticosterone ratio is low in gestation and in neonatal life (around 5.5), but this doubles within 1 wk of birth, and, by the age of 2 yr reaches the adult ratio of approximately 15:18.

The fetal steroid excretion pattern differs from the adult in the following respects. It has a relatively greater excretion of sulfurylated steroids, especially of the 16-hydroxylated series; it has a relatively increased excretion of corticosterone series; it utilizes 6β-hydroxylation and oxidation of 11β-OH steroids so that cortisol may be excreted as 6β-OH cortisone derivatives; and the reduction of the Δ^4, 3-ketone structure of cortisol is less than that of cortisone.

CONTROL OF STEROIDOGENESIS IN FETAL LIFE

Up to 20 wk of gestation, development of the fetal adrenal cortex is dependent on HCG and, after 20 wk, on ACTH from the fetal pituitary. Development of the adrenal cortex beyond the 20-wk stage is halted in anencephalic fetuses. There are data to indicate that fetal Leydig cell activity and the onset of testosterone synthesis are dependent on HCG. The bulk of placental HCG goes to the maternal compartment, but it has been shown that the HCG concentration in the fetal compartment at 11–12 wk is 30 times the threshold for physiologic response (Bruner, 1951). There is definite proof of HCG uptake by the fetal compartment (Lauritzen and Lehrmann, 1967).

It is clear that HCG and ACTH affect different enzyme systems in the adrenal of the fetus. Morphologic studies showed that ACTH given intra-amniotically induced changes in the fetal adrenals different from those induced by HCG. Chemical studies revealed that HCG in the newborn results in increased DHEA excretion, while ACTH injection resulted mainly in increased cortisol production.

OTHER ENDOCRINE CHANGES IN PREGNANCY

Both fetal and maternal endocrine glands are important in fetal development. The hypothalmic-hypophysial system is essential to development of the target endocrine glands. The thyroid in the fetus becomes active at about the twelfth week of gestation; absence of fetal thyroid function results in decreased somatic and neural maturation. Masculine differentiation is absolutely dependent on the presence of the fetal testis. The fusion and differentiation of the Wolffian system and degeneration of the Müllerian system are dependent on testicular hormones. The fetal testis is capable of synthesis of testosterone and the inception of this process precedes the differentiation of the Wolffian system.

ENDOCRINE CHANGES IN THE MATERNAL SYSTEM IN PREGNANCY

As levels of estrogens increase during the course of pregnancy, there is a parallel increase in plasma protein-bound iodine (PBI) and T_4 levels, reflecting an increase in thyroxin-binding globulin (TBG). Toward the end of pregnancy, there is normally a PBI level of around 11 $\mu g/100$ ml and T_4 is increased similarly. There are increased plasma and urinary 17-hydroxycorticosteroids during pregnancy without any evidence of hypercorticism; this is at least partly due to a progressive increase in plasma cortisol-binding globulin (CBG). This binding protects the steroid from immediate hepatic inactivation, and may be responsible at least in part for changes in the pathways in corticosteroid excretion in pregnancy. Later, high progesterone levels may displace cortisol from CBG.

ENDOCRINE CHANGES IN PARTURITION

The placenta probably has a predetermined life span (*e.g.*, the aromatization of steroid ring A decreases with placental aging). The aging placenta becomes more sensitive to the effects of neurohypophysial oxytocin, but this hormone is not absolutely necessary for fetal expulsion. All of the factors that initiate labor are not fully understood, but it is likely that decreasing levels of progesterone as well as the sensitivity to oxytocin are important initiating factors in this process. The fetal adrenals are probably involved in the timing of the gestation period, premature delivery being associated with hyperplasia, and prolonged gestation with hypoplasia, of the gland (Murphy, 1973). During delivery, the levels of 17-OHCS increase markedly, and drop sharply at the termination of labor. The excretion of HCG continues for about 1 wk after parturition, and its persistence would suggest retained placental tissue.

GESTATIONAL TROPHOBLASTIC NEOPLASTIC SYNDROMES

Gestational trophoblastic neoplasms represent a group of abnormalities of placental tissue which may arise at any time following conception (Lewis,

Gore, and Goss, 1966). According to their morphologic features, locations, and invasiveness, some of these neoplasms may precipitate early termination to the pregnancy. In others, the pregnancy may go to term, and the trophoblastic neoplasm then originates from residual retained placental tissue. The time of appearance of these tumors probably does not determine the form or severity of the process, and, therefore, does not alter the natural history to any significant extent.

Trophoblastic neoplasms represent abnormal evolution of the biologic features of trophoblast elements of the placenta. The epithelial elements of the chorionic villi may undergo myxomatous degeneration and their matrixes may become swollen. The vascular elements of the chorionic villi become compressed as a result of the swelling and the stroma become quite distended, resulting in the formation of the hydatid form of each villus.

The incidence of trophoblastic neoplasm is difficult to establish firmly because of various technical and statistical reasons, but Hertz (1972) states that, in accidental population, the incidence of hydatidiform mole is 1 in 2,000–3,000 live births. The incidence in Asiatic and African countries is apparently considerably higher. He also estimates that the frequency of further trophoblastic disease following hydatidiform mole ranges from 2–10%, with a smaller percentage presenting as choriocarcinoma. About 60% of patients with choriocarcinoma give a history of a prior molar pregnancy, and about 20% present following a term delivery. The remaining 20% of patients with choriocarcinoma may have a history of various disorders of menstrual cyclicity, including irregular periods, rare tubal pregnancy, and missed abortions.

The clinical presentation of a patient with molar pregnancy varies considerably. The patient may complain of 3–4 mo of amenorrhea associated with breast engorgement, morning sickness, urinary frequency, and lower abdominal fullness, and occasional spotting or bleeding, all suggestive of early pregnancy. Physical findings include the usual cervical signs of pregnancy, including a soft cervix and variable degrees of uterine enlargement. The ovaries are usually enlarged and cystic in about 30% of the patients. Rarely, there may be galactorrhea. A few patients may have an elevated blood pressure, proteinuria, and edema, all suggestive of early toxemia of pregnancy. Fetal heart tones are not heard. This combination of findings strongly suggests the presence of a hydatid mole. The ovarian enlargement is of special significance if it occurs in the early stages. It is strongly consistent with the presence of hydatid mole rather than of any other trophoblastic tumor.

Laboratory parameters used to assess the presence of a hydatidiform mole include the plasma or urinary levels of gonadotropins which are quantitated by biologic assay or, more conveniently, by radioimmunoassay for LH. The radioimmunoassay for serum LH is now widely used for monitoring tumor growth or regression, since the presence of tumor is reflected by amounts of gonadotropin considerably outside of the limits in normal or postmenopausal women. Research by Goldstein and Gore (1967) suggests that the human placental lactogen (HPL, somatomammotropin) may also aid in the diagnosis and followup of hydatiform mole. In pregnancy, the levels of HPL and gonadotropins correlate well, but, in the presence of hydatidiform mole, there is a disparity in the elevations of these hormones with a relatively lesser increase in HPL. Occasionally trophoblastic tumors may produce other hormonally active peptides, e.g., TSH and prolactin.

Treatment of hydatiform mole requires thorough evacuation of the uterus, followed by a dilation and curettage. Some workers claim that prophylactic chemotherapy with methotrexate or actinomycin D may reduce the frequency of malignant trophoblastic tumors, but there is no universal agreement on this point. Should the markedly elevated levels of gonadotropins persist after evacuation of the mole, then the possibility of invasive mole (chorioadenoma destruens) should be considered.

In the presence of invasive mole, the chorionic villus structure is retained, but microscopic signs of invasion into surrounding uterine structures are present. Distant spread of the process may be found in the lungs, brain, and other parts of the body. Histologic examination of these metastases reveals evidence of their origin from the chorionic villus. It is claimed that persistence of the chorionic villus pattern is good evidence that the process is benign. The clinical sequels of metastases may be serious, however, depending on their size and location. A trophoblastic embolus may produce severe morbidity and even death. Trophoblastic metastases erode blood vessels and proliferate rapidly. Therapy on this type of trophoblastic tumor requires chemotherapy with methotrexate or actinomycin D. Resolution of the process is monitored by levels of gonadotropins. It is recommended that pregnancy should be postponed for at least 1 yr during which time the improvement in gonadotropin levels is monitored.

In choriocarcinoma, there is loss of villous structure in all places of occurrence. This tumor is highly invasive, malignant, metastasizes readily, and is almost inevitably fatal unless vigorously treated. As a general rule, a malignant trophoblastic tumor free of residual villous structure carries an ominous prognosis. Plasma or urinary gonadotropins serve as excellent methods of gauging severity of this disorder. Hormone levels persist and continue to increase in the presence of a highly malignant choriocarcinoma and, if, after uterine evacuation, there is a persistent elevation of chorionic gonadotropins beyond 30–60 days, then the presence of choriocarcinoma is quite likely. These patients should be treated vigorously with chemotherapy for at least two to three courses. Rarely, hysterectomy may be adjunctive in the therapeutic regimen. The treatment regimen involves intermittent use of methotrexate, actinomycin vinblastine, and purine antagonists, along with close monitoring by serum or urine levels of chorionic gonadotropins (by radioimmunoassay for LH activity). Vigorous therapy has resulted in a relatively high cure rate.

REFERENCES

Abraham, G. E., W. D. Odell, R. S. Swerdloff, and K. Hopper. 1972. Simultaneous radioimmunoassay of plasma FSH, LH, progesterone, 17-hydroxyprogesterone, and estradiol 17-β during the menstrual cycle. J. Clin. Endocrinol. 34:312–318.

Arey, L. B. 1965. Developmental Anatomy. 7th Ed. W. B. Saunders Company, Philadelphia. Chap. 2.

Ask-Upmark, J. E. 1926. Le corps jaune est-il necessaire pour l'accomplishment physiologic de la gravidite humain? Acta Obst. et Gynec. Scandinav. 5:211.

Bruner, J. A. 1951. Distribution of chorionic gonadotropin in mother and fetus at various stages of pregnancy. J. Clin. Endocrinol. 11:360–374.

Cargille, M., J. L. Vaitukaitis, J. A. Bermudez, and G. T. Ross. 1973. Differential effect of ethinyl estradiol upon plasma FSH and LH relating to time of administration in the menstrual cycle. J. Clin. Endocrinol. 36:86–94.

Donovan, B. T., and J. J. Van Der Werff Ten Bosch. 1965. Physiology of Puberty. The Williams & Wilkins Co., Baltimore. Chap. 1.

Federman, D. D. 1967. Abnormal Sexual Development. W. B. Saunders Company, Philadelphia. pp. 1–14.

Goldenberg, R. L., E. O. Reiter, and G. T. Ross. 1973. Follicle response to exogenous gonadotropins: an estrogen mediated phenomenon. Fertil. & Steril. 24:121–125.

Goldstein, D. P., and H. Gore. 1967. Trophoblastic disease. Clin. Obst. Gynec. 10:2–31.

Gray, M. J., K. S. Strausfeld, et al. 1968. Aldosterone secretion rates in the normal menstrual cycle. J. Clin. Endocrinol. 28:1269–1275.

Hertz, R. 1972. Gestational trophoblastic neoplasm. Hospital Pract. 7:157–164.

Judd, H. L., and S. S. C. Yen. 1973. Serum androstenedione and testosterone levels during the menstrual cycle. J. Clin. Endocrinol. 36:475–481.

Lauritzen, C., and W. D. Lehrmann. Levels of chorionic gonadotropin in the newborn infant and their relationship to adrenal dehydroepiandrosterone. J. Endocrinol. 39:173–180.

Lauritzen, C., C. H. L. Shackleton, and F. L. Mitchell. 1968. The effect of exogenous human gonadotropin on steroid excretion in the newborn. Acta Endocrinol. 58:655–660.

Lewis, J., H. Gore, and D. A. Goss. 1966. Treatment of trophoblastic disease with rationale for the use of adjunctive chemotherapy at the time of indicated operation. Am. J. Obst. & Gynec. 96:710–725.

Mikhail, G. 1970. Hormone secretion by the human ovaries. Gynec. Invest. 1:5–20.

Mishell, D. R., I. H. Thorneycroft, Y. Nagata, T. Murata, and R. M. Nakamura. 1973. Serum gonadotropin and steroid patterns in early human gestation. Am. J. Obst. & Gynec. 117:631–642.

Mitchell, F. L., and C. H. L. Shackleton. 1966. The excretion of Δ^5-steroid like compounds in the newborn infant. Proceedings of the Second International Congress on Hormonal Steroids. p. 152. Excerpta Medica, Amsterdam.

Murphy, B. E. P. 1973. Does the human fetal adrenal play a role in parturition? Am. J. Obst. & Gynec. 115:521–525.

Perlroth, M. G., H. S. Marver, and D. P. Tschudy. 1965. Oral contraceptive agents and the management of acute intermittent porphyria. J. A. M. A. 194:1037–1042.

Ross, G. T., C. M. Cargille, M. B. Lipsett, P. L. Rayford, J. R. Marshall, C. A. Stott, and D. Rodbard. 1970. Pituitary and gonadal hormones in women during spontaneous and induced ovulatory cycles. Recent Progr. Hormone Res. 26:1–29.

Ryan, K. J., and Z. Petro. 1966. Steroid biosynthesis by human ovarian granulosa and thecal cells. J. Clin. Endocrinol. 26:46–52.

Villee, D. B. 1972. Development of steroidogenesis. Am. J. Med. 53:533–544.

5

Pubertal Development and Disturbances of Menarche

Puberty progresses sequentially until adult sexual characteristics are attained (Tanner, 1969; Marshall and Tanner, 1969; Root, 1973). Because there are variations in the age at which adolescence begins, the physiologic and endocrinologic progression relates more closely to the physical stages of sexual maturation. The stages of pubertal development in the female patient have been described in detail (Tanner, 1969) and are summarized in figure 5.1 in which the sequence of breast development, pubic hair growth, menarche, and skeletal growth is depicted. Because various workers have employed somewhat different criteria for description of this progression, a comparative classification is also presented in table 5.1. Ethnic and geographic considerations affect the times of appearance of sexual characteristics, but in girls in the United States, the following landmarks are recognized. The initiation of breast development is at age 10.8 yr, the appearance of pubic hair starts at about 11 yr, the onset of menstruation is between ages 12.6–12.9 yr, and the peak height velocity is achieved at around age 12 yr. A relationship has been demonstrated between body weight and time of puberty, and, in American girls, the critical weight at which adolescent maturation begins is 47.8 kg (and the height is 155 cm). This relationship may well explain the early onset of puberty in obese girls, and delayed menarche found in starving girls. The pubertal growth spurt is accompanied by changes in several physical parameters, including an increase in muscle size and numbers of cells, energy requirements, metabolic rate, carbohydrate tolerance, and water and electrolyte balance.

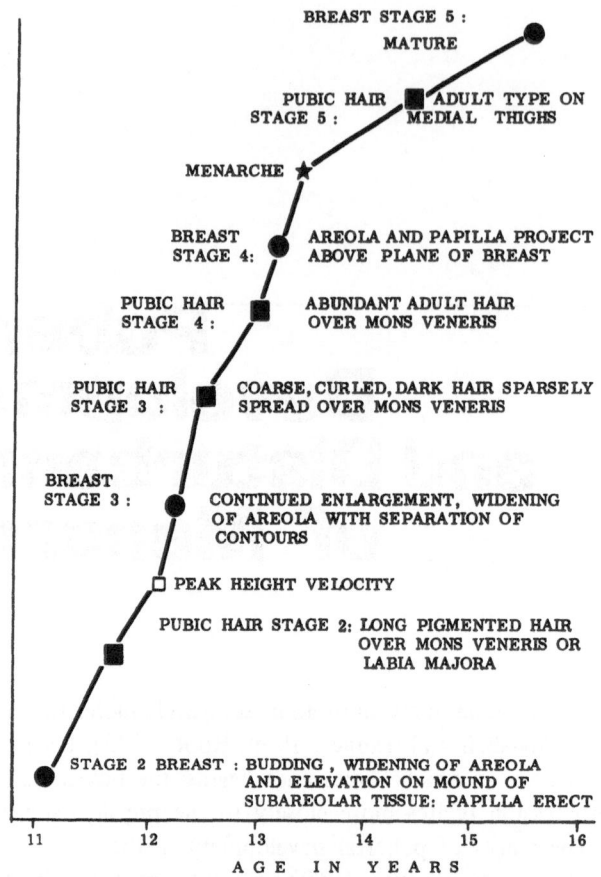

BREAST STAGE 5 :
MATURE

PUBIC HAIR ADULT TYPE ON
STAGE 5 : MEDIAL THIGHS

MENARCHE

BREAST AREOLA AND PAPILLA PROJECT
STAGE 4: ABOVE PLANE OF BREAST

PUBIC HAIR ABUNDANT ADULT HAIR
STAGE 4 : OVER MONS VENERIS

PUBIC HAIR COARSE, CURLED, DARK HAIR SPARSELY
STAGE 3 : SPREAD OVER MONS VENERIS

BREAST
STAGE 3 : CONTINUED ENLARGEMENT, WIDENING
OF AREOLA WITH SEPARATION OF
CONTOURS

PEAK HEIGHT VELOCITY

PUBIC HAIR STAGE 2: LONG PIGMENTED HAIR
OVER MONS VENERIS OR
LABIA MAJORA

STAGE 2 BREAST : BUDDING , WIDENING OF AREOLA
AND ELEVATION ON MOUND OF
SUBAREOLAR TISSUE: PAPILLA ERECT

11   12   13   14   15   16

A G E   I N   Y E A R S

Figure 5.1. Stages of female maturation. The landmark stages in pubic hair growth and breast growth are plotted against average chronologic age at time of appearance.

CHANGES IN THE HYPOTHALAMIC-PITUITARY-OVARIAN-ENDOMETRIUM AXIS AT TIME OF PUBERTY

The gonadotropic functions of the pituitary are controlled by neurohormones (releasing and inhibitory factors) secreted by hypothalamic nuclei. These nuclei are in turn controlled by neurotransmitters released by nerve endings controlled by transducer neurons. The neurohormones of the hypothalamus are secreted in the median eminence, or in other nuclei, and are stored in the median eminence until they are transported through the portal system to the anterior pituitary.

Tonic control of gonadotropin secretion resides in the median eminence, but the cyclic control center is located in the anterior hypothalamus. This center is rendered inert early in male development by exposure to androgens.

The male (tonic) or female (cyclic) control patterns of the hypothalamus in humans are established *in utero*. Control of the hypothalamic nuclei by catecholamines (dopamine, norepinephrine) and indoleamines (serotonin) is well known. A decapeptide factor extracted from this area of the hypothalamus is capable of releasing both LH and FSH from the anterior pituitary, but there are data suggesting separate LH- and FSH-releasing factors. Dopamine has been shown to release the gonadotropin releasing decapeptide GnRH. The possible relationship of the pineal organ in mediating the effects of light on the initiation of puberty was discussed in Chapter 2. There are data which suggest that melatonin from that gland may inhibit secretion of LH- and FSH-releasing factors by the hypothalamus. Of clinical significance are the observations that menarche occurs earlier in blind girls, that sexual precocity is associated with destructive pineal lesions, and that sexual infantilism has been observed in the presence of parenchymatous pineal tumors.

Estrogens commence to elicit the secretion of LH at the time of puberty. Progesterone is capable of inhibition of LH secretion by the pituitary, but FSH secretion is suppressed by a combination of progesterone and estrogen. Under the influence of FSH, multiple ovarian follicles are stimulated to development. These effects are enhanced by estrogen secreted by the theca interna (see Chapter 4). At least a twofold increase of FSH occurs between

Table 5.1. Stages of Female Pubertal Development

Clinical description	Stages	
	Johns Hopkins	University of California at San Francisco
Preadolescent	1	P-1
Breat development without growth of sexual hair	2	
Breast buddings, early labial hair growth		P-2
Breast and pubic hair development	3	
Increased breast size with palpable glandular tissue, no separation of breast contours, moderate labial hair over mons veneris		P-3
Further enlargement of breasts with projection of areola above breast plane, lateral spread of pubic hair		P-4
Adult breast size, pubic hair distribution, and menarche	4	P-5

childhood and adulthood. By radioimmunoassay studies, FSH levels were noted to increase at between ages 9–12 yr in girls. The functions of LH in the mature female are the stimulation of ovulation and the formation of corpus luteum. The role of this hormone in the prepubertal girl is not clear, however. Radioimmunoassay studies reveal that serum LH concentrations increase after 8 yr of age and during the earliest stages of puberty in girls. Serum LH levels in the postmenarchial period are significantly higher than in the pre-menarchial period. Cyclic changes in FSH and LH are achieved within the first postmenarchial year. A sleep-related increase in LH in the midpubertal female is absent in males and in prepuberty.

Plasma estradiol and estrone levels are low during childhood and increase at the time of thelarche (breast development). There is a direct correlation between chronologic age, plasma estradiol, skeletal maturation, and female adolescent development. Ovarian estrogens stimulate growth of the vagina, uterus, and endometrium. The estrogens also influence the distribution of fat deposition, skeletal maturation, and linear growth. These hormones inhibit the peripheral actions of growth hormone on growth, but the release of growth hormone in response to hypoglycemic or arginine challenges is enhanced by estrogens. Androgens are secreted by the adrenal cortex and stimulate the growth of pubic and axillary hair (adrenarche). These hormones also increase epiphyseal maturation and linear growth. Adrenal testosterone and epitestosterone are detectable in the urine of female subjects at 5–6 yr, and an increased excretion is noted at 11 yr.

Other androgens from the adrenal, including DHEA, androstenedione, and androstenediol increase several fold at the time of puberty. The plasma levels of testosterone show a less marked increase. DHEA is a weak androgen but, because of its secretion rate, may well be the most important adrenarchal androgen in the female. The mechanism of increased adrenal androgen secretion at puberty is not clear. It is possible that an inhibition of the hydroxy-steroid dehydrogenase (Δ^5, 3β-ol dehydrogenase) in the adrenal by estradiol may shunt cortical biosynthesis toward androgens, and toward DHEA in particular. The adrenal is the major source of progesterone in the preadoles-cent girl. The levels of this hormone increase slightly with age.

DISORDERS OF MENARCHE

The female infant is born with a total fund of 400,000–500,000 potential ova, of which only about 400 are destined to be released for possible fertilization. Cyclic release of ova is dependent on an intricate interplay of hypothalamic and suprahypothalamic centers, the anterior pituitary and the ovaries, as well as several peripheral factors which influence the feedback regulation of the pituitary-ovarian axis. Responsiveness of the follicular unit of the ovary is also an important factor, as there are data suggesting an age- or development-dependent refractoriness of the unit to gonadotropins. Similarly, the responses of the hypothalamic nuclei are dependent on maturation of the system. The participation of the pineal gland as a slow time clock which determines the onset of menarche has been suggested by several studies, and the occurrence of precocious puberty in male patients with pineal tumors has been cited in support of this concept. There are objections to this concept, however, and it is of special interest that pineal tumors are not frequently involved in premature development in the female (Kitay and Altschule, 1954).

The average time of menarche in the United States is at the age of 13 yr, but this is dependent on factors such as ethnic background, family history, and environmental influences. Development of secondary sexual characteristics is also dependent on similar factors and is quite variable. Disturbances of menarche are considered under the headings of delayed menarche and premature menarche.

Delayed Sexual Maturation

Delayed sexual maturation is present if thelarche has not occurred by 13 yr of age or if a period exceeding 5 yr has elapsed between thelarche and menarche. The etiologies of delayed sexual maturation in the female are presented in table 5.2 and figure 5.2.

Constitutional Delayed Menarche   In patients with constitutional delayed menarche, there is no demonstrable organic pathology. It is suggested that the retardation of sexual development probably represents a normal variation, and is correctible by time alone. The clinical manifestations seen in these patients are due to lack of sufficient amounts of estrogens for the maturation of the secondary sexual characteristics and for the initiation of uterine bleeding. This estrogen deficiency is due to an immaturity of the hypothalamic-pituitary axis so that sufficient amounts of gonadotropins (FSH and LH) are not released. In addition to genetic and familial factors in the pathogenesis of this disorder, it is likely that other factors, such as nutrition, starvation, illnesses, emotional states, as well as disturbances in other endocrine glands such as the adrenals and thyroid, are also involved. The major emphasis in the diagnostic study of patients with delayed menarche is the exclusion of organic causes of the disturbance. In constitutional delayed menarche, the bone age is compatible with the sexual age. Definitive workup is necessary if delayed menarche is accompanied by any of the following signs: absence of development of other secondary sexual characteristics, systemic disorders such as obesity, neurologic, thyroid, or adrenal diseases, psychiatric disorders, symptoms or signs of outflow tract obstruction, and the possibility of chromosomal aberration.

Table 5.2. Causes of Delayed Adolescence in Females

I. Central nervous system disorders
   A. Constitutional delayed maturation
      1. Malnutrition
   B. Congenital anomalies
      1. Hypothalamic
         a) Craniopharyngioma
         b) Absence of gonadotropin-releasing hormones
      2. Suprahypothalamic
   C. Inflammatory processes
      1. Encephalitis
      2. Granuloma
   D. Tumors
      1. Hypothalamic
      2. Pineal
   E. Trauma
II. Pituitary
   A. Congenital anomalies
      1. Aplasia
      2. Hypoplasia
      3. Absence of gonadotropins
   B. Inflammatory
      1. Granuloma
   C. Trauma
   D. Tumors
III. Gonads
   A. Congenital anomalies
      1. Turner's syndrome
      2. Gonadal dysgenesis
   B. Trauma bilateral torsion of ovarian pedicle
   C. Tumors
      1. Ovarian
         a) Bilateral neoplasms
         b) Cysts requiring oophorectomy
      2. Radiation injury
IV. Genitals
   A. Congenital anomalies
      1. Absence of uterus and/or vagina
      2. Imperforate hymen
      3. Testicular feminization
V. Systemic illnesses
   A. Cardiorespiratory
   B. Gastrointestinal
   C. Urinary
   D. Endocrine

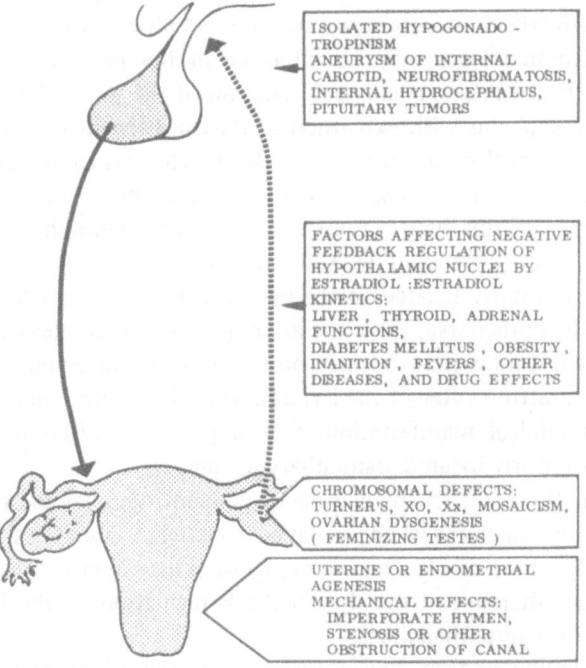

ISOLATED HYPOGONADO -
TROPINISM
ANEURYSM OF INTERNAL
CAROTID, NEUROFIBROMATOSIS,
INTERNAL HYDROCEPHALUS,
PITUITARY TUMORS

FACTORS AFFECTING NEGATIVE
FEEDBACK REGULATION OF
HYPOTHALAMIC NUCLEI BY
ESTRADIOL :ESTRADIOL
KINETICS:
LIVER , THYROID, ADRENAL
FUNCTIONS,
DIABETES MELLITUS , OBESITY ,
INANITION , FEVERS , OTHER
DISEASES, AND DRUG EFFECTS

CHROMOSOMAL DEFECTS:
TURNER'S, XO, Xx, MOSAICISM,
OVARIAN DYSGENESIS
(FEMINIZING TESTES)

UTERINE OR ENDOMETRIAL
AGENESIS
MECHANICAL DEFECTS:
 IMPERFORATE HYMEN,
 STENOSIS OR OTHER
 OBSTRUCTION OF CANAL

Figure 5.2. Etiologies of delayed sexual maturation in the female. The hypothalamic-pituitary-ovarian axis is depicted and the locations of the various etiologies are presented.

Lack of menstrual bleeding is found in patients with mechanical obstruction in the outflow tract, *e.g.*, imperforate hymen, stenosis, or other obstruction in the vaginal or cervical canals. Such obstructive phenomena are usually of a congenital nature, but may be acquired secondary to infection. These patients fail to have vaginal bleeding, but, nevertheless, may have periodic pain in the lower abdomen or in the vaginal area. On rectal examination or on palpation a fluctuant mass would suggest retained blood. Failure of menstrual flow may also occur if the endometrium is incapable of the appropriate response to estrogens and progesterone. A rare cause of such a disorder is endometrial or uterine agenesis. Acquired endometrial defects may accompany infections or mechanical damage to the endometrium.

Delayed Menarche Due to Organic Causes Insufficient or absent gonadotropin stimulation of the ovaries is associated with amenorrhea. Hypogonadotropic hypogonadism may be an isolated phenomenon or part of panhypopituitarism. Whether the defect is due to isolated gonadotropin deficiency or panhypopituitarism or is an early manifestation of evolution to the latter will depend on the anatomic location and nature of the defects. Tumors and infarction of the pituitary are frequently found causes of hypogonadotropinism since gonadotropin and growth hormone secretory activities are most sensitive to alterations in intrasellar pressures and blood flow.

Gonadotropin release may be inhibited in the presence of suprasellar disorders such as tumors, aneurysmal dilation of the internal carotid artery, internal hydrocephalus with expansion of the third ventricle, and neurofibromatosis with internal hydrocephalus. In these states, associated defects in the tropic hormones to the adrenals and thyroid are likely to occur. The most common tumor of this type is the basal suprasellar craniopharyngioma. The clinical effects are dependent on the anatomic location of the tumor. For example, an anteriorly located tumor may affect the visual fields, because of pressure on the optic nerve, as well as affect gonadotropin release. A posterior location of the tumor may infringe on release of other tropic hormones. If the appetite control center of the hypothalamus is involved, obesity becomes a prominent clinical manifestation. Sexual precocity often results from a markedly posteriorly located craniopharyngioma.

Errors in the feedback regulation of gonadotropin release may also be responsible for amenorrhea and delayed menarche. Obesity, febrile states, thyroid disease, liver disease, and drug ingestion may alter the degradation of estrogens and, thereby, affect the feedback regulation of the hypophysiotropic area of the hypothalamus.

Primary hypogonadism may occur as a congenital inherited defect, such as Turner's syndrome, which is due to an abnormal sex chromatin configuration. The most prevalent cause of this disorder is the XO complement, but the XX configuration with one abnormal X may also be responsible for abnormal gonadal development. Mosaicism in the karyotype may also be associated with gonadal defects. The typical Turner's syndrome patient is noted to be short, to have a chromatin-negative buccal smear, an XO karyotype, and high (castration) levels of FSH and LH. Associated congenital anomalies found in this syndrome include coarctation of the aorta and intestinal telangiectasia. The incidence of chromosomal abnormalities in girls 58 cm or less is relatively high, and considerably less in girls over 61 cm.

Evaluation of the patient with delayed sexual maturation requires a thorough historic review and physical evaluation. Historic information should include gestational history (maternal physical state, illnesses, drug ingestion, and nutrition), labor, the neonatal period, the occurrence of illnesses in the early neonatal period, and the patient's eating habits. The growth pattern and the sequence of sexual maturation should also be ascertained. The presence of poor nutrition or chronic illness as bases of deviations from standard growth rates should also be considered. Thorough review of the familial history is essential to determine if similar occurrences were noted previously. The routine vital signs should be obtained on physical examination. Special attention is paid to the arm span, height, and upper (crown to pubis) and lower (pubis to floor) measurements. For example, hypothyroidism is characterized by a decreased arm span and an increased upper to lower ratio. Neurologic examination is required to define abnormalities in the central nervous system. The cardiovascular, respiratory, and gastrointestinal systems are examined to rule out systemic illnesses. Sexual development is conveniently assessed by the Tanner (1969) method or similar criteria.

Gonadal dysgenesis is suspected in the phenotypic female if the following features are seen on physical examination: short stature (usually less than 58 cm), high-arched palate, webbed neck, low hairline, shield chest, poorly developed and widely spaced areolae, hypertension and decreased femoral pulse (suggesting coarctation of the aorta), multiple nevi, cubitus valgus, a palmar simian crease, and increased digital ridging. Atypical patients may show only some of the above features. A rectal and pelvic examination is essential to define the status of the uterus, the presence of an imperforate hymen, or the presence of hematocolpos.

Laboratory evaluation should include X-ray bone survey to determine bone age. A buccal smear is obtained for determination of presence of the Barr body. Additional chromosomal study may be required. In patients with constitutional delayed menarche, the retardation of bone and height ages is essentially equal. Screening laboratory tests, such as routine hemogram, urinalysis, blood glucose, serum electrolyte, chest X-ray, and tuberculin test will aid in defining the presence of chronic systemic disease.

Specific measurements of plasma FSH and LH will aid in determining the presence of pituitary or gonadal defects. Even in childhood. serum FSH and LH may be elevated in the presence of primary hypogonadism; the test is even more reliable by the age of 10 yr. Low levels of these gonadotropins are present in defects of the hypothalamic-pituitary axis. Occasional serial follow-up with FSH and LH determinations may be required to fully define a problem of delayed sexual maturation. Clomiphene stimulation test is not applicable to children since it suppresses gonadotropin release at this period. A challenge with FSH/LH-RH and measurement of FSH and LH are useful in defining the presence of hypogonadotropic hypogonadism. Tests to determine the secretion of other pituitary hormones may also be needed, e.g., TSH levels after TRF injection, GH and cortisol levels after insulin hypoglycemia (see Chapter 3).

Management of problems of delayed sexual maturation in the female depends on proper evaluation and diagnosis. In most patients with constitutional delay of maturation, only reassurance and observation are required in order to ascertain that the landmarks appear as anticipated. Behavioral problems attendant on the child's appearance may require additional management. The use of hormonal therapy is not recommended at this time however. Possibly when gonadotropin-releasing factor becomes available, such therapy may be attempted. In girls with hypogonadotropic hypogonadism, estrogen therapy is initiated at the appropriate age as ethinyl estradiol 0.02

mg daily for 21 days/mo. Within increasing age, the dose is increased, and a progestin is added as required to prevent endometrial hyperplasia. Thyroid hormone replacement is given when appropriate. In patients with hypergonadotropic hypogonadism, estrogen replacement therapy is instituted at the appropriate age. Patients with testicular feminization (chromatin negative) are reared as females, the testes are removed, and estrogen therapy is initiated at the appropriate age.

The disorders discussed above will again be considered under a discussion of the causes, pathogenesis, and management of primary amenorrhea.

Premature Menarche

As defined above, the normal age of menarche in the United States is 13 yr. Normal girls may show evidence of increased estrogens earlier however, as thelarche and pubarche (growth of pubic hair) occur by the age of 9 yr. Premature sexual development is present if cyclic uterine bleeding starts before 10 yr of age, or if thelarche and pubarche start before 8 yr. A benign disorder of precocious thelarche, without pubarche and menarche, is found in certain patients with end-organ hypersensitivity to estrogens. Isosexual precocity refers to sexual development appropriate to the phenotype of the individual; heterosexual precocity indicates sexual characteristics at variance with the patient's phenotype.

Isosexual precocity occurs more commonly in girls than in boys. The various causes of female isosexual precocity are listed in table 5.3 and figure 5.3. True sexual precocity refers to the premature activation of normal mechanisms which control the hypothalamic-pituitary-ovarian axis. Accordingly, adult levels of pituitary gonadotropins are secreted in adult sequence and the ovaries respond normally to this stimulation. A review of over 500 cases of female sexual precocity revealed that around 90% may be of a constitutional, cryptogenic, or idiopathic nature (Kitay and Altschule, 1954). Organic lesions are identifiable as the basis of true sexual precocity in the rest of the patients.

Constitutional Sexual Precocity Constitutional sexual precocity is characterized by premature release of pituitary gonadotropins in adult amounts and sequence (Van Der Werff Ten Bosch, 1969). Undoubtedly, this premature release is due to activity of the hypophysiotropic area of the hypothalamus. The reasons for the early onset of these processes are not yet clear. The gonadotropic hormones stimulate ovarian follicular activity, with increased estrogen production, ovulation, and menstruation resulting. There is premature initiation of breast development and of pubic and axillary hair. In these patients, menarche may antedate pubarche and thelarche, in contrast to individuals who develop in the normal sequence of thelarche, pubarche, and menarche. In many cases, this disorder may be of genetic origin. It has been

Table 5.3. Causes of Sexual Precocity in the Female

I. True sexual precocity
   A. Constitutional sexual precocity
   B. Precocity due to organic causes
      1. Tumors
         a) Lesions in tuber cinereum and in posterior hypothalamic area
         b) Lesions which destroy the pineal organ (rarely)
         c) Hamartoma in tuber cinereum or mamillary body (with fibers to the hypothalamus)
         d) Astrocytoma
         e) Neurofibroma
         f) Ependymoma
         g) Craniopharyngioma
         h) Suprasellar teratoma
         i) Optic glioma
      2. Nontumorous processes
         a) Encephalitis
         b) Meningitis
         c) Internal hydrocephalus
         d) Tuberous sclerosis
         e) Diffuse cerebral atrophy
         f) Trauma with cerebral involvement
         g) Mongolism and polydactylism
         h) Primary and iatrogenic hypothyroidism
         i) McCune-Albright syndrome (polyostotic or monostotic fibrous dysplasia)
         j) Corticosteroid treatment of congenital adrenocortical hyperplasia
II. Organic precocious pseudopuberty due to secretions by
   A. Ovaries
      1. Granulosa cell tumors
      2. Thecal cell tumors
      3. Follicular cysts
      4. Teratomas
      5. Chorionepithelioma
   B. Adrenal cortex
      1. Hyperplasia associated with 21-hydroxylase deficiency, 11β-hydroxylase deficiency, or Δ^5, 3β-ol-dehydrogenase (hydroxysteroid dehydrogenase) deficiency
      2. Tumors with biosynthetic defects or with overproduction of gonadal hormones
         a) Adenoma
         b) Carcinoma
   C. Ingestion or absorption of exogenous estrogens or androgens (e.g., poultry, meats, plants, ointments, creams, medications)
   D. Iatrogenic administration of human chorionic gonadotropins or androgens

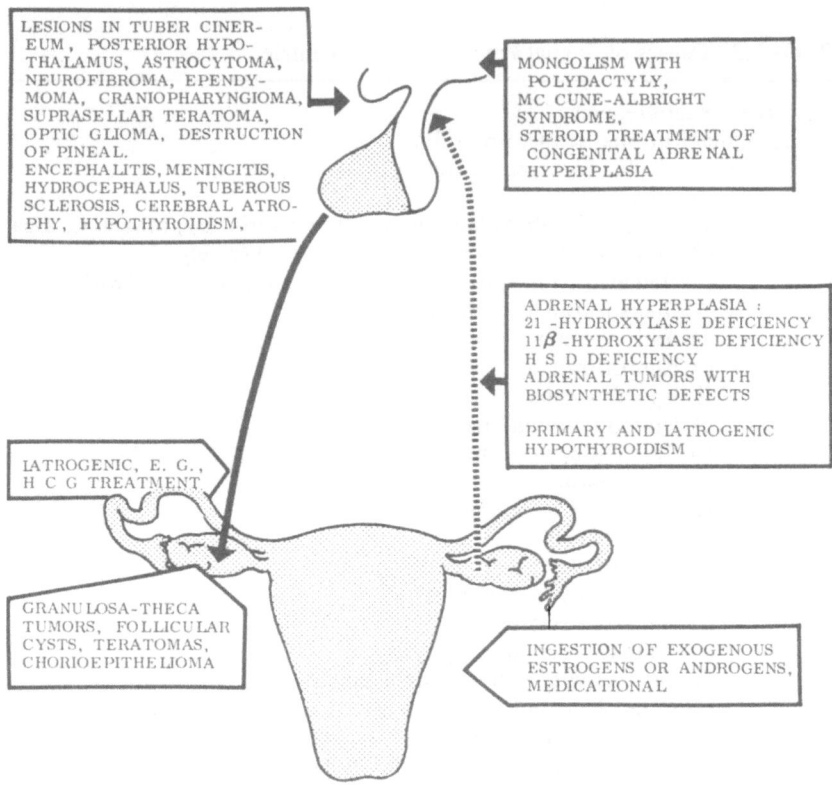

LESIONS IN TUBER CINER-
EUM, POSTERIOR HYPO-
THALAMUS, ASTROCYTOMA,
NEUROFIBROMA, EPENDY-
MOMA, CRANIOPHARYNGIOMA,
SUPRASELLAR TERATOMA,
OPTIC GLIOMA, DESTRUCTION
OF PINEAL.
ENCEPHALITIS, MENINGITIS,
HYDROCEPHALUS, TUBEROUS
SCLEROSIS, CEREBRAL ATRO-
PHY, HYPOTHYROIDISM,

MONGOLISM WITH
POLYDACTYLY,
MC CUNE-ALBRIGHT
SYNDROME,
STEROID TREATMENT OF
CONGENITAL ADRENAL
HYPERPLASIA

ADRENAL HYPERPLASIA :
21 -HYDROXYLASE DEFICIENCY
11β-HYDROXYLASE DEFICIENCY
H S D DEFICIENCY
ADRENAL TUMORS WITH
BIOSYNTHETIC DEFECTS

PRIMARY AND IATROGENIC
HYPOTHYROIDISM

IATROGENIC, E. G.,
H C G TREATMENT

GRANULOSA-THECA
TUMORS, FOLLICULAR
CYSTS, TERATOMAS,
CHORIOEPITHELIOMA

INGESTION OF EXOGENOUS
ESTROGENS OR ANDROGENS,
MEDICATIONAL

Figure 5.3. Etiologies of sexual precocity in the female are presented against the background of the hypothalamic-pituitary-adrenal axis.

suggested that a reduction of inhibitory hypothalamic influences may be etiologically related to the onset. Increased pituitary and ovarian sensitivity to the hypothalamic factors have also been considered as possible mechanisms of onset of this disorder.

Most patients with constitutional sexual precocity ovulate. The presence of ovulation effectively rules excess estrogen production independent of pituitary gonadotropin stimulation. Therefore, ectopic estrogen production from the adrenals, or exogenous estrogens, do not simulate the complete pattern of constitutional sexual precocity.

Ovulation and menstruation are due to the interplay of FSH, LH, and the gonadal hormones. All other clinical manifestations in this disorder are due to secretion of estrogens in adult amounts. Estrogens stimulate linear growth so that these patients are temporarily taller than their contemporaries, but continued growth is terminated by early estrogen-induced epiphyseal closure.

Accordingly, girls of 8 or 9 yr with constitutional sexual precocity are usually taller than their contemporaries only for a 2- to 3-yr period, and their adult height is usually below average.

The diagnostic criteria for female constitutional sexual precocity include the following: premature thelarche, pubarche, and menarche, advanced bone age, adult levels of gonadotropins and estrogens, and absence of adnexal masses in patients with normal adrenocortic and neurologic functions and a normal sella turcica. A biphasic basal body temperature is seen only in patients who ovulate and does not differentiate a granulosa cell tumor from a patient with constitutional precocity who is anovulatory. Vaginal cytology shows estrogen effects and may reveal cyclic changes in those patients who are ovulatory. Adult levels of FSH and LH with the mid-cycle surge are found in these patients. Estradiol levels follow the adult pattern also.

Precocious Puberty Due to Organic Causes Several organic lesions are responsible for premature appearance of puberty (see table 5.2). In all of those conditions, the common feature responsible for the early maturation of the pituitary-ovarian axis is a loss of the hypothalamic inhibitory influences on the sequential release of adult amounts of FSH and LH. Experimental studies have shown a clear relationship of the posterior hypothalamic lesions and the early onset of puberty, probably through disruption of the hypophysial portal circulation. It is suggested that pineal tumors may cause precocious puberty partly because of their proximity to this area. With exclusion of hypothalamic inhibitory influences by the disrupted portal system, early release of FSH and LH takes place. Hamartomas or hyperplasia in the tuber cinereum also affect these hypothalamic inhibitory influences, thus causing sexual precocity. Similar phenomena are noted in presence of astrocytoma, neurofibroma, ependymoma, craniopharyngioma, suprasellar teratoma, and optic glioma. It is difficult to differentiate patients with sexual precocity due to midbrain lesions from those with constitutional sexual precocity, unless there is X-ray evidence of an intracranial space-occupying lesion. Neurologic signs and symptoms may also be helpful in differential diagnosis.

Nontumorous processes such as encephalitis, meningitis, internal hydrocephalus, tuberous sclerosis, and diffuse cerebral atrophy are often accompanied by precocious sexual maturation through unknown mechanisms. Occasionally, intracranial trauma is followed by signs of precocious development within a period of 4–8 wk. Mongolism with polydactyly, hypothyroidism, and McCune-Albright syndrome (polyostotic or monostotic fibrous dysplasia with skin pigmentation) are frequently associated with precocious sexual development. The precocious puberty associated with primary and iatrogenic hypothyroidism has been ascribed to indiscriminate overproduction of pituitary gonadotropins, but there are experimental data which suggest that decreased gonadotropin degradation is a likely mechanism. The elevated TRF formed in primary hypothyroidism might be etiologically related to sexual precocity because of the increase in prolactin due to increased TRF.

The Silver syndrome is a form of sexual precocity which is characterized by short stature, asymmetry, and increased levels of FSH and LH. Several patients with congenital adrenocortic hyperplasia with biosynthetic defects were noted to develop true sexual precocity after suppression therapy with corticosteroids. This is probably due to a sudden rapid release of releasing factors resulting from the suppression therapy.

Organic Pseudoprecocious Puberty or Organic Precocious Pseudopuberty Premature maturation of female sexual characteristics may occur in disorders causing increased secretion of estrogens or in the presence of exogenous estrogens (fig. 5.4). This group of clinical disorders is characterized by the absence of cyclic menstrual bleeding. Uterine bleeding due to endometrial hyperplasia and sloughing may occur, but no secretory endometrial changes are seen and the bleeding is not cyclic. Ovarian disorders, such as granulosa cell tumors, thecal cell tumors, follicular cysts, teratomas, and chorionepitheliomas may secrete sufficient amounts of estrogens to stimulate pubarche and thelarche, as well as endometrial proliferation. Ovarian tumors are found in 1–2% of girls with precocity, and 75% of these are estrogen-producing tumors or cysts, including granulosa cell tumors, thecal cell tumors, thecomas, luteomas, mixed granulosa and thecal tumors, thecal lutein cysts, and follicular cysts. Tumors such as teratomas, dysgerminomas, and chorionepitheliomas may cause sexual precocity by the ectopic production of gonadotropins which induce noncyclic hyperestrogen production by the ovaries.

Sexual precocity may develop as early as the first year of life. The earliest manifestation is thelarche, followed by increased weight and height, and advanced skeletal maturation. These patients may occasionally exhibit a whitish or brownish vaginal discharge and occasional noncyclic uterine bleeding. Abdominal pain and swelling may be noted and sexual hair and acne may occur. Rectoabdominal examination (under anesthesia) often discloses the presence of a tumor. Thecal cell tumors are less frequently palpable than granulosa cell tumors.

Most granulosa cell tumors are now considered to be mixed granulosa-thecal tumors. Only 5% of this type of tumor occurs prepubertally. Thecal cell tumors are malignant in 3% of the cases. As suggested above, ovarian chorionepetheliomas and teratomas may produce gonadotropins. The finding of an abdominal mass in a girl with sexual precocity is strong evidence of an ovarian tumor. Massive levels of plasma or urinary estrogens are diagnostic of an ovarian tumor. Increased levels of chorionic gonadotropin (HCH) is evidence for a tumor of the gonadotropic type.

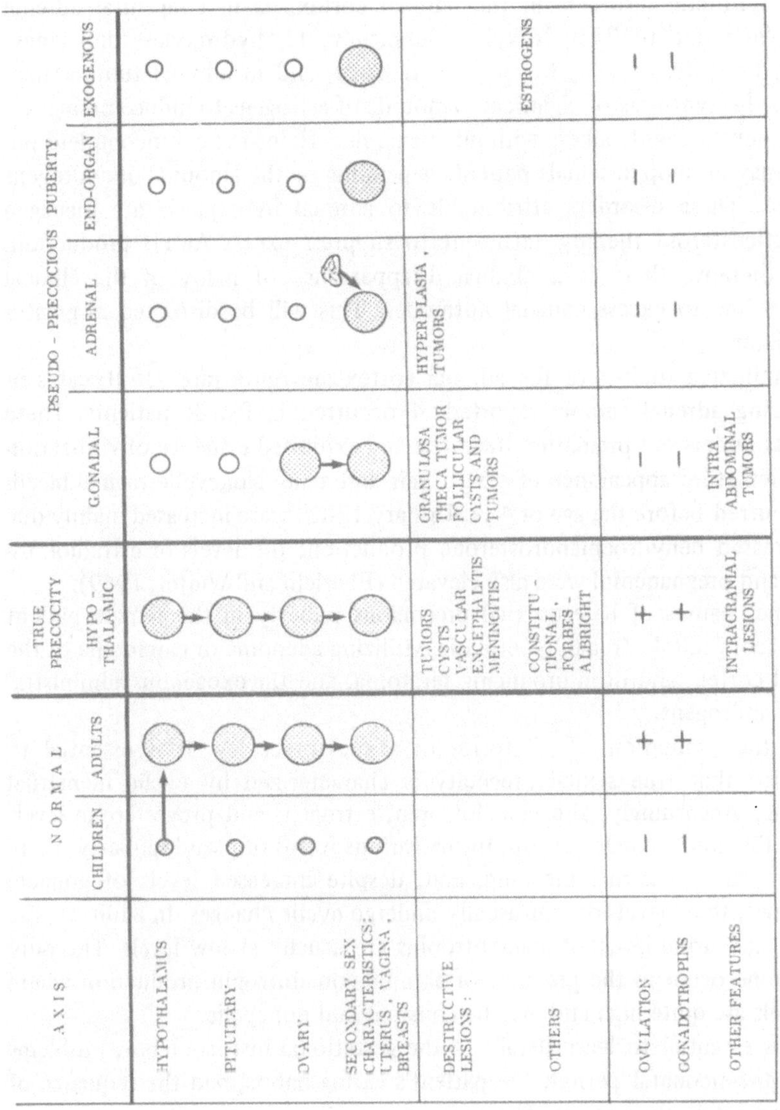

AXIS	NORMAL		TRUE PRECOCITY	PSEUDO - PRECOCIOUS PUBERTY			
	CHILDREN	ADULTS	HYPO-THALAMIC	GONADAL	ADRENAL	END-ORGAN	EXOGENOUS
HYPOTHALAMUS							
PITUITARY							
OVARY							
SECONDARY SEX CHARACTERISTICS: UTERUS, VAGINA, BREASTS							
DESTRUCTIVE LESIONS :			TUMORS CYSTS VASCULAR ENCEPHALITIS MENINGITIS	GRANULOSA THECA TUMOR FOLLICULAR CYSTS AND TUMORS	HYPERPLASIA, TUMORS		ESTROGENS
OTHERS			CONSTITU- TIONAL. FORBES - ALBRIGHT				
OVULATION	−	+	+	−	−	−	−
GONADOTROPINS	−	+	+	−	−	−	−
OTHER FEATURES			INTRACRANIAL LESIONS	INTRA- ABDOMINAL TUMORS			

Figure 5.4. Sexual precocity and pseudopubertal development are presented according to the levels of involvement. Clinical and laboratory findings in the various disorders are also depicted.

Therapeutic measures include the prompt removal of all tumors and cysts when found. Teratomas should be removed along with the uterus and adnexa because of the malignancy potential of this type of tumor. Chemotherapeutic measures may occasionally be necessary.

Biosynthetic disorders in the adrenal cortex, as in congenital adrenal hyperplasia due to 21-hydroxylase deficiency, 11β-hydroxylase deficiency, and hydroxysteroid dehydrogenase deficiency, and in adrenal tumors, may lead to the synthesis of significant amounts of estrogens to induce premature sexual development, albeit without menarche. Heterosexual incomplete puberty may develop in female patients depending on the amounts of androgens released. These disorders attributable to adrenal hyperplasia are managed by corticosteroid therapy sufficient to suppress excess ACTH production. After therapy, there is a gradual disappearance of many of the clinical features due to excess gonadal hormones. This will be discussed in greater detail later.

Feminizing tumors of the adrenal cortex are quite rare. Of 10 cases of feminizing adrenal tumors reported, 4 occurred in female patients. These patients underwent premature thelarche and exhibited evidence of virilization with premature appearance of sexual hair and acne. Noncyclic vaginal bleeding occurred before the age of 4 yr. Urinary 17-KS were increased mainly due to increased dehydroepiandrosterone production; the levels of estradiol, estrone, and pregnanediol were also elevated (Eberlein and Winter, 1969).

Other causes of heterosexual precocious puberty in the female patient include congenital adrenal hyperplasia, virilizing adenoma or carcinoma of the adrenal cortex, androgen-producing teratoma, and the exogenous administration of androgens.

In the evaluation of all forms of sexual precocity, it is essential to recognize that true sexual precocity is characterized by cyclic menstrual bleeding. Accordingly, the gonadotropin, estrogen, and progesterone levels follow the adult female pattern. In the various forms of pseudopuberty, there is no cyclic menstrual bleeding, and, despite increased levels of gonadal hormones, these levels do not usually undergo cyclic changes. In addition, the plasma and urine levels of gonadotropins are usually at low levels. The only exceptions occur in the presence of ectopic gonadotropin production where the levels are quite high and may be constant and noncyclic.

It is essential to learn details of the gestational history, labor, problems during the neonatal period, the patient's eating habits, and the sequence of development in the patient. The occurrence of illnesses as well as exposure to drugs and chemicals should be considered. If possible, data on height-weight progression should be obtained. In addition, it is essential to determine whether other family members had any similar endocrine problems. On physical examination the routine parameters of blood pressure, pulse, height, weight, head, and chest circumferences should also be ascertained. The arm span as well as upper (crown to pubis) and lower (pubis to floor) measurements should be obtained as these may be of diagnostic importance. For example, short limbs and increased upper to lower ratios are observed in patients with hypothyroidism. An adequate neurologic examination is essential to define abnormalities of the central nervous system.

The degree of sexual maturation is conveniently determined by the criteria of Tanner (1969). Evidence of estrogen effects on the breasts, areolae, and external genitals is obtained. The presence of skin manifestations of gonadal hormone effect is also ascertained, *e.g.*, presence of sebaceous glands, secretions, and acne. Certain skin manifestations that are characteristic of disease entities are also sought. For example, in the McCune-Albright syndrome, there are café au lait spots with irregular edges (coast of Maine outline). Rectal and rectoabdominal examinations, occasionally under anesthesia, may be necessary to determine the presence of intra-abdominal masses and suprarenal masses.

Skull X-rays are necessary to ascertain the presence of increased intracranial pressure on the space-occupying lesions; careful attention is directed to abnormal calcifications and to enlargement of the sella turcica. On occasion, air encephalography and electroencephalography may be necessary to determine the presence of intracranial abnormalities. Skeletal maturation is determined by bone surveys, and the presence of monostotic or polyostotic fibrous dysplasia may also be determined by such survey. Patients with true sexual precocity show markedly advanced bone age. In patients with premature thelarche, the bone age is consistent with the chronologic age. There may be a slight advance in normal bone age in patients with premature adrenarche, but a definite retardation is seen in patients with hypothyroidism. When necessary, pelvic peritoneography or laparoscopy may permit visualization of the ovaries and pelvic adnexa. Arteriography, perirenal air insufflation, and intravenous pyelography may be helpful in identifying adrenal masses in patients showing evidence of precocious development.

Plasma and urine FSH and LH levels are elevated in true sexual precocity and exhibit the adult cyclic pattern. This pattern is seen in constitutional sexual precocity as well as in patients with organic true sexual precocity. Therefore, these levels do not provide complete differentiation of these etiologies. Plasma 17β-estradiol levels are markedly elevated in girls with ovarian granulosa-thecal tumors. Pregnanediol in the urine is increased in patients with thecal ovarian tumors, in patients with gonadotropin-producing tumors, as well as in patients with true sexual precocity during the luteal phase of the cycles.

Urinary 17-KS levels are elevated in patients with virilizing adrenal hyperplasia, and in patients with adrenocortic tumors, and this measurement is especially useful in the diagnostic workup of female heterosexual precocity. Urinary pregnanetriol levels are elevated in adrenal hyperplasia associated with 21-hydroxylase deficiency. Tetrahydrodesoxycortisol levels are increased in the 11β-hydroxylase deficiency form of congenital adrenal hyperplasia. Elevated levels of 17-KS and 17-ketogenic steroids in congenital adrenocortical hyperplasia are suppressed by exogenous corticosteroids such as cortisol and dexamethasone. This suppression test is, therefore, useful in this disorder. Plasma testosterone levels are elevated in various forms of isosexual and heterosexual precocity. The suppressibility of increased levels with exogenous dexamethasone is often helpful in the differential diagnosis of these disorders.

Management of Female Sexual Precocity The management of these disorders depends on the nature of the underlying defect. As indicated previously, constitutional sexual precocity represents the adult pattern occurring prematurely. The natural history of the disorder is, nevertheless, quite variable. After the diagnosis is established, and organic causes of the disorder are ruled out, it is essential that the patient be observed for a 6- to 12-mo period before any therapy is instituted. Periodic followup studies should be obtained on bone age, epiphyseal closure, and development of the external secondary sexual characteristics. In the absence of marked progression, continued observation is recommended. The major indications for therapy are rapid progression of bone growth and impending epiphyseal closure. General management also should include advice to the parents and teachers that the patient should be protected from possible sexual abuse. In the face of rapid progression of sexual maturation, the progestin compound depo-medroxyprogesterone (Depo-provera) is employed for its antigonadotropin effect. The drug is administered in doses of 100–200 mg intramuscularly every 2–4 wk. This regimen is followed by decreased levels of FSH and LH, marked estrogen diminution, cessation of menses, and decrease in breast size and pelvic bone. Amenorrhea then supervenes. The duration of treatment is determined by these parameters as well as by bone age changes. Unfortunately, in most patients, the bone age progression and epiphyseal closure may continue unabated, presumably because of delay in institution of therapy. If, however, an abatement of this process is noted, this therapy is continued until the patient achieves an adequate height. Side effects of the drug include increased appetite, fluid retention, weight gain, suppression of adrenocortical function, prolonged inhibition of the hypothalamic-pituitary axis, and possible chromosomal damage. Therefore, the physician must be very cautious in prescribing this drug for long periods of time. The phenothiazine drugs have been tried in the management of this disorder, but are not recommended as they suppress growth hormone secretion as well as that of FSH and LH.

In patients with central nervous system lesions, surgical intervention may be necessary. In patients with sexual precocity due to hypothyroidism, adequate thyroid replacement therapy is followed by regression of sexual development.

It is anticipated that antagonists to the hypothalamic releasing factors may be helpful in the management of these patients in the future.

Patients with pseudoprecocity due to ectopic production of gonadotropins should be treated surgically. Depending on the malignancy potential of the particular tumor, chemotherapy may be indicated occasionally as an adjunct. In patients with pseudopuberty secondary to adrenal production or to other lesions, removal of the excess gonadal hormones may occasionally be followed by an abrupt increase of gonadotropins and may induce true sexual precocity.

Premature thelarche and adrenarche do not require definitive medical therapy. Girls with premature thelarche should wear loose-fitting clothing in order to de-emphasize their contours.

REFERENCES

Eberlein, W. R., and J. S. D. Winter. 1969. Adrenal tumors in childhood *In* L. I. Gardner (ed.), Endocrine and Genetic Diseases of Childhood, pp. 437–442. W. B. Saunders Company, Philadelphia.

Kitay, J. I., and M. D. Altschule. 1954. Gonadal changes associated with pineal tumors. *In* The Pineal Gland, Chapter 18. Harvard University Press, Cambridge.

Marshall, W. A., and J. M. Tanner. 1969. Variations in pattern of pubertal changes in girls. Arch. Dis. Child. 44:291–303.

Root, A. W. 1973. Endocrinology of puberty. J. Pediat. 83:1–19; 83:187–200.

Tanner, J. M. 1969. Growth and endocrinology of the adolescent. *In* L. I. Gardner (ed.), Endocrine and Genetic Diseases of Childhood, pp. 14–69. W. B. Saunders Company, Philadelphia.

Van Der Werff Ten Bosch, J. J. 1969. Isosexual precocity. *In* L. I. Gardner (ed.), Endocrine and Genetic Diseases of Childhood, pp. 554–564. W. B. Saunders Company, Philadelphia.

6
Amenorrhea

Amenorrhea, the absence or cessation of menstrual bleeding, is a clinical symptom which may result from several underlying physiologic and mechanical aberrations (Philip et al, 1965; Hertz et al., 1966; Abraham et al., 1972). Primary amenorrhea is a failure of menarche to occur by the age of 18 yr. Secondary amenorrhea is the cessation of menses for a period longer than 3 mo in patients who have previously menstruated. Some patients may undergo menstrual cyclicity and uterine bleeding without external appearance of blood; this condition is correctly termed **cryptomenorrhea**, and should not be confused with primary or secondary amenorrhea. Physiologic amenorrhea, the absence of menses before puberty, after the menopause, and during pregnancy and lactation, is a normal phenomenon.

As described in Chapter 4, the pattern of regular menstrual cyclicity is dependent on an intricate interplay between the vaginal tract, uterus, ovaries, and the pituitary-ovarian axis as controlled by the hypophysiotropic area of the hypothalamus. Several factors affect the operation of this axis, such as the adrenals, thyroid, liver function, nutrition, drug ingestion, and pathologic states. It is useful to analyze problems of menstrual cyclicity with these anatomic areas in mind (figs. 6.1 and 6.2).

The outflow of uterine secretions and bleeding are dependent on the patency of the vaginal tract and cervical canal. Congenital disorders, as well as infections, may cause stenosis in these tracts with consequent cryptomenorrhea. The most frequently encountered cause of cryptomenorrhea is probably the imperforate hymen. Patients with this disorder complain of monthly attacks of lower abdominal or back pain. Physical examination often reveals the presence of hematocolpos or hematometra in addition to an obviously intact hymen. Therapy consists of hymenectomy and drainage of the secretions. Vaginal agenesis with or without uterine agenesis are also causes of primary amenorrhea. These patients exhibit all the other secondary female sexual characteristics. Diagnosis is usually made by physical examination and by dye studies to determine patency of these organs. These conditions may be treated surgically when appropriate. The outlook for marital relationships

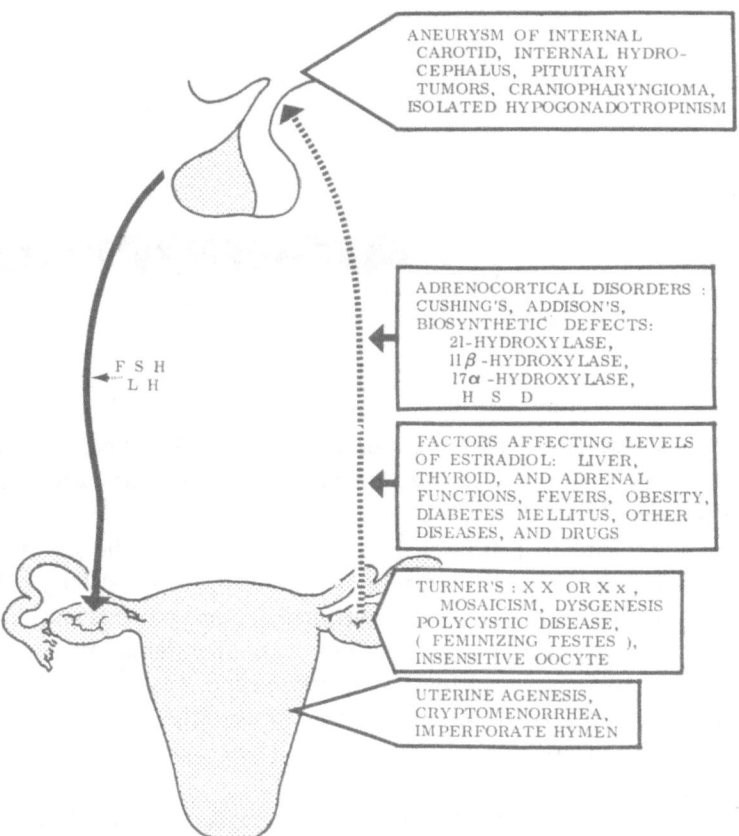

Figure 6.1. Causes of primary amenorrhea are depicted against the hypothalamic-pituitary-ovarian axis and feedback circuit to elucidate mechanisms of the various disorders. The participation of extragonadal and peripheral factors on activity of the circuit is emphasized. See text for further discussion.

is good but that of procreation is absent. Damage by trauma, infection, or radiation to the endometrium may render this tissue incapable of responding to estrogens and progesterone. Vigorous curettage may result in scarring of this layer, as in Asherman's disease. Tuberculous involvement of the endometrium is not uncommon as a cause of this disorder.

PRIMARY AMENORRHEA

One of the more common causes of primary amenorrhea is a defect in ovarian function caused by abnormal chromosomal constitution, as is found in Turner's syndrome with the chromosomal constitution 45-XO, or presence of an abnormal X chromosome (45-Xx), with resultant gonadal dysgenesis. In addition to primary amenorrhea, these patients exhibit several associated clinical features including: (1) sexual infantilism with scanty pubic hair and poorly developed breasts; (2) short stature with dubitus valgus; (3) webbed neck, low hairline at the back of the neck, and low set ears; (4) ocular abnormalities which may include nystagmus, strabismus, and ptosis; (5) a protuberant sternum with shield-shaped chest; (6) mental retardation (in some); (7) ovarian agenesis or dysgenesis (streaked gonads on laparoscopy); (8) lack of estrogen effect on vaginal smear; (9) low plasma and urine estrogens; (10) high urine and plasma FSH and LH; (11) X-ray findings of shortening of the fourth metacarpal and metatarsal bones, and deformity of the medial tibial condyle; (12) associated cardiovascular anomalies, including coarctation of the aorta which may occur in 25% of the patients; and (13) associated urinary tract abnormalities in 50% (most frequently, horseshoe kidney). Considerably less frequently, primary amenorrhea is associated

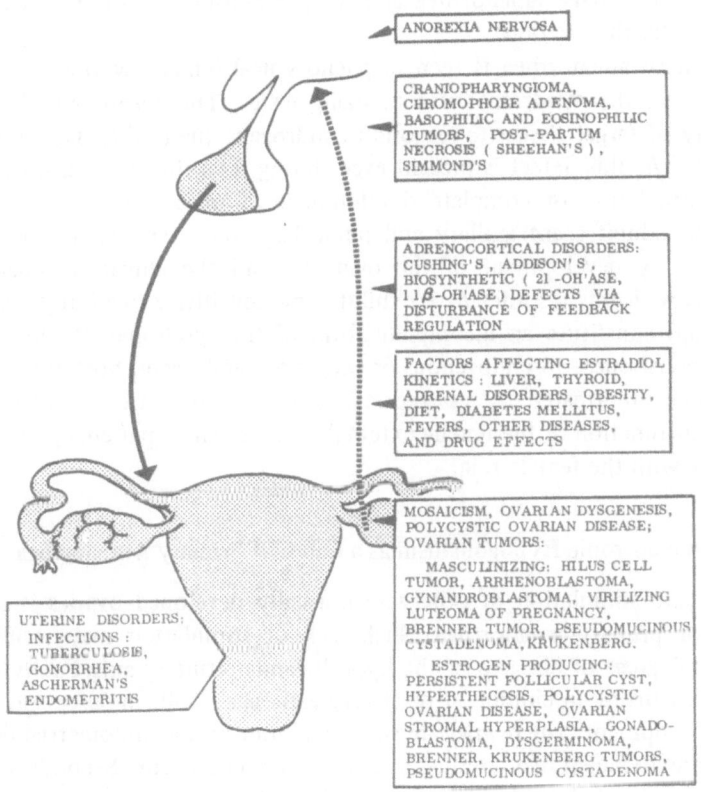

ANOREXIA NERVOSA

CRANIOPHARYNGIOMA, CHROMOPHOBE ADENOMA, BASOPHILIC AND EOSINOPHILIC TUMORS, POST-PARTUM NECROSIS (SHEEHAN'S), SIMMOND'S

ADRENOCORTICAL DISORDERS: CUSHING'S , ADDISON'S , BIOSYNTHETIC (21 -OH'ASE, 11β-OH'ASE) DEFECTS VIA DISTURBANCE OF FEEDBACK REGULATION

FACTORS AFFECTING ESTRADIOL KINETICS : LIVER, THYROID, ADRENAL DISORDERS, OBESITY, DIET, DIABETES MELLITUS, FEVERS, OTHER DISEASES, AND DRUG EFFECTS

MOSAICISM, OVARIAN DYSGENESIS, POLYCYSTIC OVARIAN DISEASE; OVARIAN TUMORS:

MASCULINIZING: HILUS CELL TUMOR, ARRHENOBLASTOMA, GYNANDROBLASTOMA, VIRILIZING LUTEOMA OF PREGNANCY, BRENNER TUMOR, PSEUDOMUCINOUS CYSTADENOMA, KRUKENBERG.

ESTROGEN PRODUCING: PERSISTENT FOLLICULAR CYST, HYPERTHECOSIS, POLYCYSTIC OVARIAN DISEASE, OVARIAN STROMAL HYPERPLASIA, GONADO-BLASTOMA, DYSGERMINOMA, BRENNER, KRUKENBERG TUMORS, PSEUDOMUCINOUS CYSTADENOMA

UTERINE DISORDERS: INFECTIONS : TUBERCULOSIS, GONORRHEA, ASCHERMAN'S ENDOMETRITIS

Figure 6.2. Causes of secondary amenorrhea. See explanation to figure 6.1.

with polycystic ovarian disease, but this etiology is more likely in secondary amenorrhea.

Primary amenorrhea can result from disorders in the adrenal cortex with biosynthetic defects. Three forms of these biosynthetic defects are responsible for the overproduction of gonadal hormones (as in 21-hydroxylase, 11β-hydroxylase, and hydroxysterioid dehydrogenase deficiencies) which interfere with the negative feedback control of gonadotropin release. Primary amenorrhea along with sexual infantilism are found in 17α-hydroxylase deficiency which affects both the adrenals and the gonads. Some of these defects may also be the basis of secondary amenorrhea and will, therefore, be discussed in greater detail under that section.

Disorders of the thyroid may also be responsible for primary amenorrhea. Thyroid hormones are involved in the maturation of the hypothalamic-pituitary-ovarian axis, and exert a permissive effect on the actions of the gonadal hormones. In addition, thyroid hormones affect the hepatic metabolism of estrogens and, accordingly, influence the negative feedback control of the hypothalamic-pituitary axis by estradiol. These disorders may also be the basis of secondary amenorrhea and will, therefore, be considered in more detail under that section.

Primary amenorrhea is seen in phenotypical females who are chromatin negative in the syndrome of feminizing testes. This disorder is due to an inability of target tissues to respond to androgens due to their lack of cytosol receptor. As this defect is present even during fetal life, there is no Wolffian duct stimulation or complete development of male characteristics. These patients exhibit scant axillary and pubic hair, the uterus is absent, there is rudimentary development of the oviducts, and the clitoris is small. Rare patients with this disorder may exhibit some sensitivity to androgen stimulation, and constitute an incomplete form of the syndrome. Because of the nonresponsiveness to endogenous or exogenous androgens, both forms of this syndrome are treated by castration and exogenous estrogen sufficient to maintain function of the female external genitals. These patients permanently identify with the female role.

Hypogonadotropic Hypogonadism as a Cause of Primary Amenorrhea

Inadequate stimulation of otherwise normally developed ovaries is a major cause of primary amenorrhea. Such lack of stimulation may result from varying degrees of diseases of the hypothalamic-pituitary axis. Panhypopituitarism occurring in childhood or at very early age results in defects in growth and development. The ovaries are small, and uterine and endometrial development are deficient, so uterine bleeding does not occur. Secondary sexual characteristics fail to develop as a result of lack of stimulation of ovarian function by gonadotropins. In childhood, the most common cause of hypogonadotropinism is craniopharyngioma derived from Rathke's pouch (which is of suprasellar location). Degree of involvement of the pituitary depends on the location of the tumor. A posterior location of the tumor may involve the median eminence, and panhypopituitarism usually results. A relatively anterior location is frequently associated with hypogonadotropinism. Local pressure may also result in encroachment of the optic chiasm, with consequent visual field defects. The secretion of gonadotropins and growth hormone are most sensitive to alterations in blood flow and pressures in the intrasellar compartment. Nontumorous disorders, such as aneurysm of the internal carotid and internal hydrocephalus with expansion of the third ventricle, may also decrease gonadotropin release. In such situations, decreased corticotropic and thyrotropic functions, as well as hypogonadotropinism, also occur. If the lesions affect the hypothalamic appetite center, hypothalamic obesity results.

Isolated hypogonadotropinism is fairly common and may be due to localized hypothalamic-pituitary disease, as well as to errors in the feedback regulation of this system resulting from systemic disease, obesity, and emotional trauma. Diagnostic workup of these various causes of primary amenorrhea will be discussed after consideration of secondary amenorrhea (see fig. 6.1).

SECONDARY AMENORRHEA

Secondary amenorrhea refers to the cessation of menstrual bleeding in a patient who has previously menstruated. For practical purposes, this abnormality is considered significant if the patient has not menstruated for a period equivalent to three or four normal cycles. The onset of this disorder may be quite abrupt, or may follow a period of oligomenorrhea (menses of diminishing frequency). The physiologic secondary amenorrheas are quite common and are seen in pregnancy, the puerperium, the postmenarchial period, the premenopause, and, in an irreversible state, the menopause.

There are several nonhormonal causes of secondary amenorrhea. These include obstructive lesions, such as cervical stenosis which obstructs drainage of uterine secretions. Such stenosis may result from cauterization procedures, conization, irradiation, chemical burns, and infections. Endocervical malignancy may decrease the caliber of the cervical canal. Endometrial disease is often the basis of secondary amenorrhea. Destruction of the endometrium may follow irradiation and infections such as tuberculous endometritis. Asherman's syndrome designates endometrial sclerosis and synechiae following vigorous curettage. Endometrial atrophy and ovarian inactivity may follow the use of long-acting progestational agents, perhaps as a result of prolonged suppression of gonadotropins.

The forms of secondary amenorrhea due to hormonal aberrations may be due to disorders of the hypothalamic-pituitary-ovarian axis and of the feedback control of this axis. In this context, it is essential to also consider nonpituitary and ovarian factors which affect the control of the axis by ambient levels of gonadal hormones, or by suprahypothalamic factors which influence the axis (fig. 6.2).

Secondary Amenorrhea Due to Ovarian Disorders

Amenorrhea caused by disturbed ovarian function may be due to either an inability of the ovary to respond to appropriate stimulation or to an abnormality in hormone production of the ovaries, with resultant disruption of the feedback regulation of the hypothalamic-ovarian axis.

Diminished ovarian production of hormones prior to the age of 40 yr is responsible for an irreversible form of secondary amenorrhea in premature ovarian senescence. This disorder is characterized by decreased levels of gonadal hormones and increased levels of gonadotropins. The basis of this disorder is not clear. Premature ovarian failure is also found in patients with the XXX chromosomal constitution. Sexual infantilism is found in this disorder, but not in patients with premature ovarian senescence. Although most patients with gonadal dysgenesis exhibit primary amenorrhea, a number of such patients with gonadal dysgenesis, who are chromatin positive, may have secondary amenorrhea.

Polycystic Ovarian Syndrome

The syndrome of polycystic ovaries was originally described by Stein and Leventhal (1935) to be characterized by menstrual abnormalities, oligomenorrhea or amenorrhea, obesity, virilization or hirsutism in one-half of the patients, and infertility. The ovaries in these patients were enlarged, thickened, and pale, and contained numerous cystic follicles beneath the capsule. Microscopic examination revealed fibrosis of the cortical stroma and areas of hyalinization, with evidence of unusual activity of the theca interna cells with luteinization in the cystic follicles. Similar features have been described in the ovaries with adrenocortic disorders and in experimental animals exposed to increased androgens. Ovaries in this syndrome rarely reveal evidence of ovulation, and corpora lutea are rarely found. This finding is confirmed by the finding of proliferative hyperplastic endometrium. Many patients with polycystic ovarian disease have since been studied, and it is now apparent that this syndrome represents a rather wide spectrum of abnormalities characterized by increased androgen secretion by the ovaries, and perhaps of the adrenal, and inappropriate levels of FSH and LH. Obesity is no longer considered an essential finding in the Stein-Leventhal syndrome, and neither are acne and virilization, despite the demonstrated increased levels of androgens in such patients.

The etiology of the polycystic ovarian syndrome is not known, but considerable biochemical data suggest that the hypothalamic-pituitary-ovarian axis feedback regulation is disturbed. It is not clear whether the primary defect is in the hypothalamus or in the ovaries. It is possible that the feedback circuit is disturbed by inappropriate overproduction of ovarian androgens (and estrogens) with resultant inappropriate FSH and LH levels. It has been suggested that the gonadotropins are secreted only in a tonic fashion in this disorder, but other data reveal inappropriately high levels of LH in these patients. One concept of the etiology of this syndrome suggests excessive sensitivity of the ovaries to gonadotropins, resulting in the growth of numerous follicles. With only partial development, these follicles become cystic. Stromal hyperplasia and luteinization of the theca result from the persistent inappropriate elevation of LH (Yen et al., 1970). It has also been suggested that the basic error in this syndrome is secondary to a hypothalamic defect, whereby the nuclei in the tonic area release the neurohormones in a constant, rather than cyclic, manner. Inertia of the cyclic center is also a possible mechanism, albeit different from the fetal origin of a similar inertia in male subjects. The histologic characteristics of the ovaries are consistent with constant stimulation, and it is possible that this persistent estrogen production is responsible for noncyclic tonic low-level release of LH.

There are considerable amounts of data indicating that the abnormal level of androgens such as testosterone is a major factor in the genesis of the polycystic ovarian syndrome. Polycystic ovarian disease is found in patients with virilizing adrenocortical hyperplasia, as well as in animals given excess androgens. A possible defect in the conversion of androstenedione to estrogen has been suggested as the basis of increased androstenedione and, subsequently, of testosterone, in this syndrome. However, it is also possible that the total amount of partially stimulated follicles may be responsible for excessive androgen production. Although both androstenedione and testosterone levels in the plasma of Stein-Leventhal patients are elevated, kinetic studies suggest that the excess plasma testosterone is derived from a precursor other than androstenedione. Patients with Stein-Leventhal syndrome have been shown to have plasma testosterone levels of around 0.33 mg/100 ml (range 0.25–0.42 mg/100 ml) compared with the level in normal women of 0.050 mg/100 ml (Lloyd et al., 1966). Studies by Kirschner and Bardin (1972) revealed significantly elevated levels of testosterone in this syndrome, with an even greater increase of androstenedione. Gambrell, Greenblatt, and Mahesh (1973) provided data confirming earlier concepts of three patterns of androgen secretion in the Stein-Leventhal syndrome, those with primarily an ovarian source of androgens, those with excessive adrenal secretion of androgens, and those with combined ovarian and adrenal androgen excess. Indeed, these authors suggest that the persistent LH secretion may well be secondary to the altered levels of androgens from those sources. On the other hand, Taymor and Barnard (1962) suggest that excess LH may stimulate both adrenal and ovarian androgen secretion and, therefore, LH excretion data should not be used as a diagnostic tool to differentiate between adrenal and ovarian types of the polycystic ovarian disease. These authors also concluded that the absence of progesterone may well be the basis of the persistent (and inappropriate) LH secretion. If there is indeed a defect in the Δ^5, 3β-ol dehydrogenase (hydroxysteroid dehydrogenase) system in this disorder, then decreased progesterone production is not unexpected (see Chapter 4).

The clinical observation that wedge resection of the ovaries of patients with Stein-Leventhal syndrome is followed by resumption of menstrual cycles in some patients, albeit even temporarily, has been cited as proof of decrease of the elevated androgen production with the resultant restitution of the feedback regulation of the hypothalamic-pituitary ovarian axis. Several studies revealed decreased androgen levels in the plasma after wedge resection Laboratory studies in the diagnosis of this disorder will be presented later in this chapter. The significant clinical features of Stein-Leventhal syndrome (sclerocystic or polycystic ovarian disease) include the following: (1) secondary amenorrhea or oligomenorrhea usually follows months or years of irregular anovulatory cycles; (2) the onset may be gradual over a number of years; (3) menorrhagia may occur in about 15% of the cases; (4) the patients are usually infertile; (5) obesity is common but not universal; (6) hirsutism, clitoromegaly, and other evidence of virilization occur frequently; (7) immature female development is occasionally found; (8) the ovaries are bilaterally enlarged in all cases; (9) multiple ovarian cysts are seen within a dense fibrous stroma with the absence of corpora lutea or albicantia; (10) failure of ovulation is evidenced by a monophasic basal temperature chart; and (11) there is an increased incidence of hyperplasia and carcinoma of the endometrium in these patients.

Ovarian Lesions with Excessive Hormone Production

Secondary amenorrhea may result from disturbance of the hypothalamic-pituitary regulatory mechanism by excessive production of androgenic or estrogenic hormones by the ovaries. The androgen-producing lesions induce changes of defeminization prior to masculinization. Accordingly, amenorrhea is preceded by oligomenorrhea, and acne, hirsutism, clitoromegaly, male-type alopecia, beard formation, and deepening of the voice are preceded by loss of breast size and feminine contours. But, because the major manifestations are due to excessive androgens, the findings of defeminization are not present in all cases. The masculinizing ovarian tumors are arrhenoblastoma (Sertoli-Leydig tumor), hilus cell tumor, virilizing luteoma of pregnancy, gynadroblastoma, pseudomucinous cystadenoma, the Brenner tumor, and certain metastatic tumors which may have steroidogenic potential.

  Arrhenoblastoma (Sertoli-Leydig cell tumor), although rare, is the most common androgenic ovarian tumor. It occurs most commonly during the childbearing period with most of the over 250 reported cases appearing between ages 25–45 yr. These tumors are unilateral in most patients and are usually smooth but may occasionally be lobulated, cystic, or solid with a diameter usually between 0.5 and 15 cm. Three histologic types of arrhenoblastoma have been reported, the tubular form of Peck (which has the appearance of a tubular adenoma), the atypical form (which has imperfect tubules and irregular columns of cells), and the undifferentiated or sarcomatoid type (which has very few tubular patterns). The cell types may be either cuboidal or columnar in the tubules or glands, spindle-shaped or epithelioid cells in the sarcomatous areas, and large polygonal cells with central nuclei and abundant cytoplasm in the Leydig cells.

The major clinical features in patients with arrhenoblastoma are: (1) virilization with hirsutism, temporal baldness, acne, clitoromegaly, male-type musculature and voice, but these adrogenic stigmata are not absolutely required for the diagnosis; (2) breast atrophy; (3) palpable ovarian mass in 60% of cases; (4) amenorrhea preceded by oligomenorrhea and infertility; and (5) regression of the above findings after extirpation of the tumor. The laboratory features of special interest in this disorder will be discussed later.

Hilus cell tumor of the ovary is a rare benign tumor which occurs most commonly in menopausal and postmenopausal women. These tumors are composed of pure highly differentiated Leydig cells and are formed in association with stomal and hilar cell hyperplasia. These tumors secrete testosterone, and the urinary 17-KS in these patients is often normal. The major clinical feature is virilization of relatively long standing. This masculinization includes receding hairline, hirsutism, clitoromegaly, and deepening of the voice. Rarely, some patients exhibit features suggestive of excess production of adrenal-type steroids, including the 11β-hydroxylated androgens and mineralocorticoids. However, these findings are ascribed to rare lipoid cell tumors of the ovaries.

Virilizing luteoma of pregnancy is regarded as an inactive thecal cell tumor which is stimulated by the high levels of HCG in pregnancy. Recent studies (Lipssett and Kirschner, 1970) revealed that there is significant androgen production by this tumor, sufficient to induce defeminization, oligomenorrhea, hirsutism, changes in hair distribution to the male type, clitoromegaly, and deepening of the voice. In some patients with this disorder, there is spontaneous disappearance of the clinical manifestations within weeks or months after delivery. These tumors are often confused with adrenal rest tumors; some authors suggest that virilizing luteomas should be considered as a variety of arrhenoblastoma, but the spontaneous recovery of the virilization in many patients would be argument against this grouping.

Gynandroblastoma or Sertoli-Leydig cell tumor is a rare tumor which contains a mixture of various histologic elements suggestive of both granulosa cell tumor and arrhenoblastoma. The tumor represents a fairly undifferentiated gonadal mesenchyme which retains the bisexual potency of the fetal gonad. Accordingly, these tumors have the ability to synthesize androstenedione as well as testosterone and estradiol. The masculinizing potency of the tumor is probably greater than the estrogen effect, but there may be variable mixtures of the effects. Virilization, hirsutism, and clitoromegaly may be combined with irregular menstrual bleeding. In some cases, hypermenorrhea is the presenting complaint. The size of the tumors vary considerably (ranging from 1–20 cm in diameter). The histologic pattern is a mixture of various elements suggesting both granulosa cell tumor and arrhenoblastoma. It is, therefore, very difficult to make a definitive diagnosis of gynadroblastoma. This tumor may possess a similar malignancy potential as that of arrhenoblastoma.

The Brenner tumor, a relatively rare tumor, is found mainly in postmenopausal women and is probably derived from the ovarian stroma. This tumor is usually hormonally inactive, but it may possess the ability for androgen production consistent with its stromal origin. The visual presenting manifestation is of an abdominal mass.

Pseudomucinous cystadenomas probably contain significant stromal elements and are occasionally the source of androgen production.

Metastatic tumors from the gastrointestinal tract to the ovaries (Krukenberg tumors) may, in rare cases, induce marked proliferation and luteinization of the ovarian stroma with resultant androgen production.

Estrogen-producing lesions in the ovaries are characterized by presence of active stromal elements. The clinical manifestations may be local, such as the presence of an adnexal mass, or hormonal. The types of hyperestrogen effects are dependent on the age at which the elevated hormones occur. In prepubertal girls, the major manifestations are of sexual pseudoprecocity consisting of premature thelarche, pubarche, increased uterine size, and endometrial hyperplasia. These patients do not ovulate, as cyclic changes in gonadotropin release do not occur. In patients in the reproductive years, varying degrees of oligomenorrhea are followed by amenorrhea and absence of ovulation. In postmenopausal patients, the major effects of increased estrogens are uterine bleeding secondary to endometrial hyperplasia, as well as increase in breast size. These patients may appear younger than their chronologic ages if the hyperestrogen effects begin sufficiently early. These patients lack the typical postmenopausal uterine and vaginal mucosal atrophic changes. Excessive estrogen production by the ovaries may occur in the following nonneoplastic disorders: persistent follicular cyst, variants of polycystic ovaries, hyperthecosis, and ovarian stromal hyperplasia. The neoplastic disorders responsible for excessive estrogen production are: granulosa-thecal tumors, tumors with active stromal components (Brenner tumors, pseudomucinous, cystadenoma, and Krukenberg tumors) which are metastatic from the gastrointestinal tract to the ovaries, dysgerminoma, gonadoblastoma, and, in rare instances, teratoma.

Hyperthecosis consists of elements of both excessive estrogen and androgen. It has been suggested that the disorder may represent an eventual evolution into a masculinizing syndrome. The initial hyperestrogen effects include irregular menses, followed by oligomenorrhea, and possibly progressing to amenorrhea. The subsequent androgenic effects include: sterility, hirsutism and temporal hair recession, uterine and endometrial atrophy, clitoromegaly, and breast atrophy.

Granulosal stromal hyperplasia may also be a basis of hyperestrogenism. There is a diffuse or nodular thickening of the ovarian cortex with a diminution of the number of ova and follicles. Excessive estrogen secretion is manifested by atypical uterine bleeding and breast enlargement.

Granulosa-thecal tumors are derived from the germinal epithelium and wall of the Graafian follicle. It has been suggested that the origin of this type of tumor is related to the loss of ovum with aging of the follicular wall. Continued gonadotropic stimulation (*e.g.,* in menopause) of the cell elements is presumed to be responsible for tumor development. Because of the presence of both granulosal and thecal elements, it has been suggested that these tumors be termed feminizing mesenchymomas. They constitute 4–9% of all ovarian neoplasms and are distributed as follows: granulosa cell, 17.5%; granulosa-thecal cell, 15%; and thecal cell, 67.5%. These tumors may occur at any age, but the granulosa cell type is usually found postmenopausally with extremely few occurances in the prepubertal period. Hormonal activity depends on the particular cell type in the tumor, and the clinical manifestations of hyperestrogenism vary according to the patient's age. These manifestations are most strikingly observed in the prepubertal child as precocious puberty with adult female contour, breast growth, presence of axillary and pubic hair, enlargement of the internal and external genitals, occurrence of anovulatory bleeding, hyperplastic endometrium, and estrogenic vaginal smear. In the postpubertal era, the major clinical manifestations of increased estrogens are irregular menses and suppressed ovulation, eventually resulting in total secondary amenorrhea. The postmenopausal patient with this tumor exhibits irregular uterine bleeding and breast enlargement and may appear younger than her chronologic age. Local manifestations of tumor growth include presence of an abdominal mass and pressure symptoms; ascites and hydrothorax are rarely found. Occasionally torsion of the ovarian pedicle may result in infarction of the gland. It is essential that the estrogen effects of this type of tumor in the prepubertal age be differentiated from those associated with constitutional sexual precocity (discussed in Chapter 5). In the reproductive period, menstrual irregularity and the presence of a solid adnexal mass should suggest a feminizing neoplasm. In the postmenopausal period, any sign of increased estrogen effect is important, and this in the presence of an adnexal mass should strongly suggest this type of neoplasm.

The Brenner tumor, which has been described previously, is most likely to occur postmenopausally. The growth rate of this lesion is quite slow. Hormonal production leads to uterine bleeding, and the patients may appear younger than their chronologic age. Local manifestations include an intra-abdominal tumor mass and occasionally ascites; hydrothorax is more commonly found.

The Krukenberg tumor is usually a secondary ovarian lesion which has metastasized from the gastrointestinal tract by lymphatic spread. The primary source is usually the stomach, but the large bowel and breasts may occasionally be sites of origin. It is difficult to differentiate these lesions from primary ovarian tumors as the ovarian contour is usually retained despite the metastatic process. These tumors may often have the appearance of granulosa-thecal tumors or of arrhenoblastoma. Estrogen production which may occur rarely is manifested by irregular uterine bleeding and breast development.

Dysgerminoma is probably derived from primordial germ cells prior to differentiation into definitive sex cells. Accordingly, male differentiation of these cells results in arrhenoblastoma, while female differentiation results in origin of a granulosa-thecal tumor. These tumors do not produce steroid hormones (androgens or estrogens), but there is a high level of production of HCG. This gonadotropin stimulates steroid production by the contralateral ovary. The presence of HCG in a female patient with a solid ovarian tumor is, therefore, quite suggestive of a dysgerminoma. Clinical manifestations in the prepubertal female patient are increased maturation and growth with uterine bleeding. In the adult, the changes are similar to those seen in pregnancy, breast enlargement, colostrum production from the nipples, and hypomenorrhea or amenorrhea. Occasionally excessive flow may occur, however. Metastasis from the tumor to the lungs results in respiratory symptoms.

The tumor is usually unilateral and may be either quite small (3 cm in diameter) or sufficiently large to fill the abdomen. The tumor is round or ovoid and the surface is either smooth or covered by a fibrous capsule which may later disappear. The microscopic characteristics include large polygonal cells with clear cytoplasm and a large central nucleus. Alveolar arrangements of cells are separated by fibrous strands. The cells usually show considerable mitotic activity. The giant cell appearance is easily confused with tuberculosis. Metastasis via lymphatic spread or by contiguity may occur in the omentum, liver, spleen, kidneys, gallbladder, pancreas, lungs, heart, thyroid, gland, and thymus.

The gonadoblastoma is similar in several respects to dysgerminoma and, in addition, displays the presence of calcification. This tumor may occur in intersex individuals, and the contralateral gonad may be a dysgenetic ovary or a testis. The uterus and one or both Fallopian tubes are usually present.

Amenorrhea Due to Adrenocortical Disorders

The various disorders of the adrenal cortex associated with amenorrhea are discussed in greater detail in Chapter 10. Adrenocortical hyperfunction may release gonadal hormones which interfere with the feedback regulation of the hypothalamic-pituitary-ovarian axis, with consequent disturbance of menstrual cyclicity. In Cushing's syndrome and Cushing's disease, the major hormonal excess is in cortisol, but, in case of excess production of gonadal-type steroids, the adrenogenital syndrome is seen. The clinical manifestations include secondary amenorrhea or, rarely, primary amenorrhea (in childhood forms). In the adult, the onset may be insidious and, in childhood, may be congenital or gradual. Major characteristics of hypercortisolemia are fatiguability and weakness, hypertension, centripetal redistribution of fat leading to moon facies, cervicodorsal fat pad and truncal obesity, hypokalemic alkalosis (10-20%), glucose intolerance (90%), depolymerized subcutaneous connective tissue with appearance of striae which appear bluish or purplish because of erythrocytosis, and osteoporosis and its consequences. The manifestations of excess androgens include acne, hirsutism and virilization, clitoromegaly, and amenorrhea. In adrenocortical hypofunction, there is considerable weakness, fatiguability, and inanition. Amenorrhea is found in approximately 30% of patients with idiopathic primary adrenocortical insufficiency. This high correlation is possibly due to autoimmune disorders affecting the adrenals and the gonads. In tuberculous adrenal insufficiency, the prevalence of amenorrhea is considerably less and is possibly secondary to inanition.

The production of excessive amounts of adrenal androgens and estrogens in several of the biosynthetic defects associated with adrenocortical hyperplasia influence the feedback regulation of the hypothalamic-pituitary-ovarian axis and, thereby, disturb menstrual cyclicity. The clinical, chemical, and laboratory diagnostic features of these disorders are described in detail in Chapter 10. These disorders are usually due to congenital defects in certain adrenocortical enzymes, but postpubertal acquired forms are also described (Prunty and Brooks, 1960; Bacchus, 1968), although this concept is now questioned (Kirschner, Zucker, and Jespersen, 1974). In all forms of virilizing adrenocortical hyperplasia, as well as in the form associated with sexual infantilism, there is a relative decrease in cortisol secretion. As a consequence, marked increases in ACTH release are found. Stimulation of adrenal hormone synthesis up to the biochemical block results in the massive overproduction of biosynthetic intermediates biologically active and inactive. Virilization, hypertrichosis, hirsutism, deepening of the voice, alterations in muscle and bony pelvic development are all effects of increased secretion of androgens. Amenorrhea results from feedback inhibition of the hypothalamic nuclei by estradiol released from the adrenals or derived from excess adrenal androgen production. The most common adrenocortical biosynthetic defect is 21-hydroxylase deficiency. This disorder in the female is characterized by virilization, clitoromegaly, hirsutism, and primary amenorrhea. The complete form of the defect is characterized by sodium loss, hyperkalemia, and hypotension because of the absence of synthesis of aldosterone or other mineralocorticoids. Deficiency of the enzyme 11β-hydroxylase is characterized by the virilizing changes described above, as well as by hypertension and hypokalemic alkalosis because of the increased accumulation of the 11-deoxy compound desoxycorticosterone. Deficiency of the adrenocortical enzyme hydroxysteroid dehydrogenase (Δ^5, 3β-ol dehydrogenase) is the basis of accumulation of the compound DHEA, which is a weak androgen. The deficiency of the 17α-hydroxylase enzyme occurs in the adrenals and ovaries and is characterized by the occurrence of sexual infantilism (hypogonadism) because of an inability to produce the substrate 17-hydroxypregnenolene, which is essential in the production of androgens and estrogens. Patients with this disorder also exhibit hypertension and hypokalemic alkalosis due to accumulation of the non-17-α-hydroxylated series such as corticosterone and desoxycorticosterone which have mineralocorticoid activity.

Amenorrhea Secondary to Thyroid Disorders

Disorders of the thyroid are discussed in greater detail in Chapter 10. Menstrual cyclicity may be profoundly disturbed in thyroid disease. In hyperfunction states (Graves' disease, Plummer's disease), in addition to the generalized effects due to hypermetabolism, there is a prominent disturbance in menstruation. This is at least in part secondary to altered degradation of estrogens and estradiol-estrone-estriol partition and a consequent disturbance of feedback regulation of gonadotropin release. In addition to the secondary amenorrhea, the clinical features of hyperthyroidism are: (1) nervousness, restlessness, and irritability; (2) weight loss despite a good appetite, although weight gain may be found early; (3) hyperdefecation and occasionally diarrhea; (4) soft, smooth, and silky hair structure; (5) increased perspiration, smooth, moist, and warm skin, occasionally with palmar erythema and onycholysis of fingernails; (6) fine tremors of outstretched fingers and tongue, with increased deep tendon reflexes; (7) exophthalmos, lid-lag or globe-lag, stare, widened palpebral fissures, and opthalmoplegia; (8) palpably enlarged thyroid gland (diffuse, with bruit, in Graves' disease, and nodular in Plummer's disease); (9) muscle weakness, with myopathy in some cases; (10) tachycardia, increased pulse pressure, atrial arrhythmias, and, occasionally, congestive heart failure; (11) pretibial myxedema; and (12) characteristic laboratory data.

Primary hypothyroidism is characterized by menometrorrhagia, but oligomenorrhea occurs occasionally. In hypothyroidism secondary to pituitary insufficiency, amenorrhea is the rule. Systemic features of hypothyroidism include: (1) increased sensitivity to cold; (2) typical facies with dull expression, thickened large features, and puffy eyelids; (3) hypomentation, poor memory; (4) constipation and flatulence; (5) diminished sweating, rough, dry skin, brittle nails, coarse and dry hair, and alopecia of outer third of eyebrows; (6) low hoarse voice and slow halting speech; (7) bradycardia,

hypotension, distant heart sounds, and, occasionally, pericardial effusion;
(8) delayed relaxation phase of the deep tendon reflexes; (9) anemia (in
50%); (10) peripheral neuropathy and paresthesias, carpal tunnel syndrome,
with motor and sensory disturbances in hands; and (11) characteristic laboratory findings (Chapter 9).

Secondary Amenorrhea Due to Hypogonadotropic Hypogonadism

Several suprahypothalamic, hypothalamic, and pituitary lesions may cause
decreased secretion, or altered sequence of release, of the gonadotropic
hormones FSH and LH. These disorders may be due to infections, traumatic,
infiltrative, or neoplastic bases. In most cases, the pituitary hypogonadotropinism is associated with decreases in other pituitary hormones, as in
panhypopituitarism. But there are now several reports of isolated gonadotropin deficiency as cause of primary and secondary amenorrhea.

Damage of the entire anterior pituitary by sepsis or embolism is the basis
of one form of panhypopituitarism known as Simmond's disease. A form of
panhypopituitarism (Sheehan's syndrome) is due to postpartum pituitary
necrosis secondary to obstetric shock. The pituitary gland is hypervascular
and engorged in the pregnant woman and it is, therefore, quite susceptible to
decreases in blood supply, such as may occur in postpartum shock, hemorrhage, infection, and hypofibrinogenemia. Secondary vasospasm of the arterial supply of the pituitary and the pituitary stalk results in infarction and
necrosis. This disorder may rarely be seen even in otherwise normal pregnancies. The clinical features of Sheehan's syndrome are described in greater
detail in another section and are summarized here. Patients with this disorder
exhibit weakness, fatiguability, and increased sensitivity to cold; apathy,
depression, and somnolence; appearance of premature aging; increased susceptibility to infections; thinning of hair and the lateral third of the eyebrows; dry skin with yellowish discoloration; atrophy of the vaginal mucosa,
uterus, and cervix; frigidity and loss of libido; failure of lactation; atrophy of
vaginal mucosa, uterus, and cervix; anemia, hypotension, and bradycardia.

Several tumors may be responsible for hypopituitarism. Of tumors of the
pituitary itself, the most common is the chromophobe adenoma: less common are the basophilic and eosinophilic tumors. Craniopharyngioma may
occur superior to the pituitary. Hypothalamic tumors may also affect pituitary function depending on the nuclei involved in the process. In all of the
situations listed above, decreased gonadotropic hormone secretion occurs,
despite the fact that specific types of tumors may produce excessive amounts
of the other pituitary hormones. For example, certain chromophobe adenomas have been found to produce significant amounts of TSH, GH, and ACTH;
eosinophilic tumors produce GH; and basophilic tumors produce ACTH. In
addition to the generalized sequels of these tumors, there are significant local

manifestations of the presence of the neoplasms such as headaches, visual field defects, oculomotor palsy, and occasionally stupors, comas, or convulsions. The clinical manifestations of these tumors will include disturbances in menstrual cyclicity in addition to the effects of the other pituitary hormones released. The features are described in greater detail in Chapter 3. Amenorrhea and ovarian failure may result from isolated deficiencies of the gonadotropic hormones. In these disorders, the clinical manifestations relative to disturbances in the other pituitary hormones are absent.

Several suprahypothalamic factors influence the activity of the pituitary-ovarian axis and may be responsible for amenorrhea and other disturbances of the menstrual cycle and reproductive functions. Emotional disturbances associated with marital and domestic problems, fear of pregnancy, physical and emotional trauma, and altered sleep rhythm may affect the actions of transducer neurons and transmitters on the hypothalamic nuclei and, thereby, influence the release of their neurohormones. This complex of disorders is often covered by the term emotional amenorrhea.

Amenorrhea Due to Other Causes

Several other disorders may directly or indirectly affect the hypothalamic-pituitary-ovarian-endometrial axis and, thereby, disturb menstrual cyclicity. Patients with anorexia nervosa may exhibit secondary amenorrhea as a prominent manifestation. In these patients, there is a psychogenic aversion to food. The consequent inanition is undoubtedly the basis of abnormal gonadotropin release, but it is probable that the turnover of gonadal hormones is altered with subsequent disturbance in the feedback regulation of the hypothalamic-pituitary-ovarian axis. The clinical features in this state include variable degrees of emaciation, occasional nausea and vomiting, and many somatic hysterical complaints such as globus hystericus, dysphagia, and epigastric fullness; delusions and phobias relative to food; depression; constipation; hypotension and bradycardia occasionally; fine generalized hypertrichosis (rarely); anemia and hypoproteinemia probably secondary to inanition, ovarian atrophy, or hypotrophy; low or absent FSH and LH and low plasma and urine estrogens, and normal parameters of adrenal and thyroid functions. GH may be increased or normal.

Alocholism with cirrhosis of the liver is a rather frequent basis of amenorrhea. Undoubtedly alterations in the partition of estrone-estradiol-estriol in the circulation results from acute and chronic disturbances in hepatic degradative functions. This results in altered feedback control of menstrual cyclicity. In addition, the frequent protein malnutrition found in these patients may be responsible for abnormal synthesis or release of gonadotropic hormones. Other causes of abnormal liver functions include posthepatitic cirrhosis, biliary cirrhosis, chronic right-sided heart failure, hemochromatosis, Wilson's disease, infectious (schistosomiasis) cirrhosis, primary cirrhosis, as well as fatty metamorphosis due to obesity, dietary inadequacies, and drug effects.

Infections with associated systemic manifestations (*e.g.*, tuberculosis) may affect gonadotropin production by inanition or by alteration in the feedback regulation of the hypothalamic nuclei by disturbed estrogen metabolism (*e.g.*, in febrile states).

PROCEDURES IN DIAGNOSIS OF AMENORRHEA

Defining the basis of amenorrhea most efficiently requires cognizance of the various links in the chain of control of the ovaries, starting in the central nervous system with ultimate affect on the endometrium (Bacchus, 1972). Biologic effects on other organ systems, *e.g.*, breasts and hair growth, may also be utilized to assay effects of hormone production by the ovaries. Amenorrhea problems are, therefore, conveniently analyzed systematically by testing of the major levels which contribute to the menstrual cycle. Accordingly, activities of the endometrium and vaginal mucosa, the functional components of the ovaries, the anterior pituitary, the hypophysiotropic area of the hypothalamus, and suprahypothalamic factors are assessed in a sequential pattern utilizing both clinical and laboratory parameters. Etiologies of cryptomenorrhea, such as mechanical defects in the endometrium, cervical canal, and vaginal canal, are not considered in this analysis. These problems may be readily diagnosed by physical examination and occasionally by radiographic techniques.

It is essential to recognize that amenorrhea is itself only a symptom and not a diagnosis. Since this symptom may reflect relatively benign as well as severe life-threatening disorders, it is important that the patient be thoroughly evaluated to rule out the latter group of diseases. Each patient should have a complete history and physical examination. Such procedure should provide information on the presence of neurologic, thyroid, or adrenal abnormalities, or possible presence of neoplasms, infections, and degenerative and systemic diseases. In addition, the presence or absence of gonadal hormonal effects is ascertained (*e.g.*, development of breasts, pubic hair, vaginal mucosa and secretions, and clitoral development). Clinical judgment should determine the laboratory procedures which are required for further delineation of the pathologic process. Based on such considerations, it is possible to group patients according to the presence of certain clinical stigmata. Accordingly, the following categories of disorders may be established (table 6.1): (1) patients with normal secondary sexual characteristics; (2) patients with ambiguous genitals; (3) patients with hirsutism; (4) patients with no secondary female sexual characteristics; and (5) patients with galactorrhea. Before con-

Table 6 1. Amenorrheic Disorders Classified According to Associated Clinical Findings

Level of involvement	Normal secondary sexual characteristics	Mild hirsutism	Ambiguous genitalia	No secondary sexual characteristics
Suprahypothalamic	Psychogenic	Psychogenic stress		Psychogenic
Hypothalamic	Hypothalamic dysfunction	Cushing's disease stress (?)		Hypothalamic dysfunction; delayed puberty
Pituitary	Panhypopituitarism; isolated hypogonadotropinism	Cushing's disease		Panhypopituitarism; isolated hypogonadotropinism
Gonad	Mosaic gonadal dysgenesis, premature ovarian senescence, polycystic ovaries (S-L) (testicular feminization)	Polycystic ovaries (S-L)	Male pseudohermaphroditism, female pseudohermaphroditism, mixed gonadal dysgenesis, true hermaphroditism	Gonadal agenesis, insensitive oocyte syndrome; pure dysgenesis; mosaic dysgenesis; 17 α-hydroxylase deficiency
Adrenal	Mild 17 α-hydroxylase deficiency	Adrenal hyperplasia with 21-hydroxylase, 11β-hydroxylase deficiency, Cushing's syndrome, adenoma, carcinoma, or hyperplasia	Congenital adrenal hyperplasia with C 21-hydroxylase deficiency, 11β-hydroxylase deficiency, HSD-deficiency	Complete 17α-hydroxylase deficiency
Uterus	Uterine agenesis; endometrial abnormality, Ascherman's disease endometritis			
Vagina	Vaginal agenesis; imperforate hymen			

sidering the procedures for differential diagnosis of the various disorders responsible for the above overt clinical manifestations, a discussion of procedures for evaluating the various levels of the axis responsible for cyclic ovarian function will be presented. These procedures have been described in detail by Bacchus (1972).

Amenorrhea Due to Disorders of the Ovaries

Hypergonadotropic Hypogonadism Ovarian hormone production is mirrored quite faithfully by the responsive endometrium. Endometrial responses during different phases of the menstrual cycle are detailed in Chapter 4, as are disorders which prevent endometrial responses to ovarian hormones; these include Asherman's syndrome, endometrial fibrosis following infections or chemical trauma, or the rare, unexplained absence of endometrial tissue.

Simple clinical procedures useful in assessment of ovarian hormonal functions include: (1) basal body temperature; (2) vaginal cytology; (3) cervical mucus ferning; (4) the progesterone withdrawal test; and (5) endometrial biopsy.

(1) **Basal** body temperature elevations of 0.5–1°F following a period of daily lower temperatures represent an effect of the elevated progesterone secretion by the corpus luteum which is formed after the process of ovulation. Failure of this biphasic temperature pattern is strongly suggestive of anovulation.

(2) **Vaginal** cytology, like endometrial cellular changes, reflects the actions of ovarian hormones. In addition, this simple procedure may reveal atypical cells, as well as changes of neoplastic disease.

(3) **Cervical** mucus examination provides information as to whether ovulation has occurred. A disappearance of the characteristic ferning pattern of cervical mucus is seen at the time of ovulation; a persistent ferning pattern reflects continued estrogen effect. For this test, a drop of cervical mucus is allowed to dry on a glass slide and then is examined under the microscope. Absence of ferning is indicative of progesterone effect or pregnancy.

(4) The progesterone withdrawal test provides information as to whether the endometrium was previously primed with estrogen. If bleeding occurs after withdrawal of progesterone, then it may be assumed that the endometrium was previously primed with estrogen or previously exposed to at least some estrogen. For the test, progesterone, or a synthetic progestational agent, is administered by intramuscular injection of 50–100 mg for 2 successive days. Withdrawal bleeding within 2–8 days after the second injection is the normal response and reflects estrogen priming of the endometrium. Alternatively, progesterone may be administered orally as 5–10 mg daily for 3 days. Absence of withdrawal bleeding is noted in pregnancy or in patients with estrogen deficiency.

(5) The purpose of the endometrial biopsy is to determine whether there are changes in ovarian hormone secretions. As discussed in Chapter 4, there are characteristic cytologic and histologic findings which correlate quite well with the amounts, types, and duration of secretion of the ovarian hormones. Accordingly, sharp ovarian biopsy specimens are often employed for endometrial dating. In the workup of amenorrhea, the finding of secretory changes in a patient who did not receive exogenous progesterone is diagnostic of progesterone effect, and, therefore, of prior ovulation. For practical purposes, it is useful to obtain three separate endometrial biopsy specimens at 2-wk intervals. This sequence should be sufficient for defining the presence of cyclic changes in ovarian function. Absence of secretory changes in all three specimens obtained in the above protocol would be consistent with an absence of ovarian cyclic activity. A recent report suggests that specimens of endometrium adequate for dating may be obtained much more simply by use of the Gravlee jet washer (Ansari and Cowdrey, 1974). This method of obtaining endometrial tissue is quite reliable in screening for atypical or neoplastic cells, but has not been extensively employed for endometrial dating.

Application of the above tests provides information both on endometrial responsiveness and ovarian cyclic activity. Obviously, normal responses in all the procedures are expected in normal individuals. Abnormal responses are consistent with noncyclic ovarian activity. A supplementary test that is quite useful in patients who did not have bleeding after progesterone withdrawal is the administration of an estrogenic substance for 20 days prior to progesterone therapy. Estinyl estradiol, 0.05 mg twice daily, is given for 20 days, after which the progesterone is administered as above. The occurrence of withdrawal bleeding after this regimen would be consistent with ovarian estrogen deficiency since exogenous estrogen corrected this defect. Absence of endometrial sloughing and withdrawal bleeding would suggest either endometrial nonresponsiveness or inadequate doses of the hormones.

If the above procedures suggest ovarian insufficiency, then the most helpful procedure to confirm this diagnosis is the determination of plasma (or urine) levels of FSH and LH. Elevated levels of these gonadotropins are expected to occur in primary ovarian insufficiency and should prompt studies to determine the etiology of the failure. Low levels of these gonadotropins in light of the above findings would be strongly indicative of pituitary insufficiency.

Amenorrhea Due to Hypogonadotropic Hypogonadism

Data obtained by the above procedures should indicate whether amenorrhea is due to an endometrial or an ovarian defect. As pointed out above, a primary ovarian defect, through the negative feedback circuit, is associated with elevated levels of FSH and LH, *i.e.*, hypergonadotropic hypogonadism. The presence of normal or low levels of gonadotropins, despite the ascertained hypoestrogenism, is consistent with a defect in the pituitary or the hypothalamic-pituitary axis, *e.g.*, hypogonadotropic hypogonadism. Delineation of disorders at this terminus of the hypothalamus-to-ovarian axis is possible by application of challenges to this axis by either clomiphene or Gn-RF (FSH-LHRH). Significant elevations of these gonadotropins in the plasma reflect the integrity of the nuclei as well as of gonadotrope cells of the anterior pituitary. Failure of elevations in FSH and LH may be due to either a defect in the hypothalamic nuclei or in the specific pituitary gonadotrope cells. To perform this test, clomiphene is given orally at the dose level of 150–200 mg daily for 7 days. Plasma FSH and LH are measured before and on the termination of the clomiphene challenge. Patients with intact hypothalamic-pituitary function exhibit significant elevations in FSH and LH. Lack of a significant elevation would suggest either a hypothalamic defect or failure of the pituitary gonadotrope cells.

The FSH-LH-releasing factor challenge is more specifically a test for pituitary gonadotropic function. The lack of a significant rise in plasma FSH and LH after a challenge with the releasing factor is indicative of deficiency at this level of the hypothalamic-ovarian axis. For this test 50–150 μg synthetic LHRH is infused intravenously over a 10-sec period. Plasma samples are obtained at −10 min, 0, 30, 60, 120, and 180 min after the infusion, and the levels of FSH and LH are measured by radioimmunoassay. Patients with normal pituitary gonadotropic functions exhibit a 5- to 10-fold elevation of LH and a less marked elevation of FSH at the time of peak response which is at the 15- to 30-min interval. Patients with panhypopituitarism fail to show significant rises in these gonadotropins after the challenge. Some patients with isolated hypogonadotropinism exhibit significant rises in LH (up to 3-fold) with essentially normal responses of plasma FSH. These data have been interpreted as indicating that isolated gonadotropin deficiency may well represent primarily a hypothalamic disorder, *i.e.*, a deficiency of the gonadotropin-releasing hormone (Zarate et al., 1973*a*; Zarate et al., 1973*b*).

Because hypogonadotropinism is often part of a more generalized hypofunction of the pituitary, it is essential that diagnosis of an isolated defect should not be made unless integrity of the other functions of the anterior pituitary is ascertained. Pituitary secretion of growth hormone is usually assessed by quantitating plasma growth hormone after a challenge of insulin-induced hypoglycemia, of arginine infusion, and, more recently, of L-dopa. Pituitary ACTH secretory capacity is assessed by cortisol elevations after the hypoglycemic challenge as above, after vasopressin challenge, or after the administration of metyrapone. These tests require the presence of intact adrenocortical tissue. The pituitary secretion of TSH is assessed by quantitation of plasma TSH after challenge with TRF.

Combined challenge for the assessment of anterior pituitary responsiveness may also be employed (Harsoulis et al., 1974). In this procedure, the patients are studied in the fasting state with the test commencing at 9:00 to 10:00 A.M. Regular insulin is administered intravenously (0.05–0.3 units/kg body weight) and followed immediately by a mixture of 200–500 μg of TRF and 100 μg of LH-FSH-RF in 5 ml of sterile water. Blood samples are obtained at 0 time, 30, 60, 90, and 120 min for quantitation of glucose, growth hormone, and cortisol. TSH, FSH, and LH levels are determined at the 0-, 20-, and 60-min intervals. The results obtained by this combined procedure were essentially similar to those obtained by the tests done separately. Normal subjects exhibit significant elevations in GH (values reaching $>$ 10 ng/ml by 60 min, with mean values around 120 ng/ml), cortisol (values at least 7 μg/100 ml greater than baseline, or a 3- to 4-fold increase by 1 hr), TSH (at least a 4-fold increase by 20 min), FSH (at least a doubling by the 20- to 60-min sampling times), and LH (at least a 2- to 4-fold increase by the 20- to 60-min sampling times). Patients with panhypopituitarism fail to show significant increases in these hormones after the combined challenge. Patients with isolated hypogonadotropinism exhibit normal GH, TSH, and cortisol responses, with partial increases in FSH and LH. Other considerations in this disorder are presented above.

Amenorrhea Due to Adrenocortical Disorders

Amenorrheic disorders secondary to diseases of the adrenal cortex may be suspected from clinical manifestations of either increased or decreased levels of adrenal hormones or their biosynthetic intermediates. As described above, Cushing's syndrome is characterized by hypercortisolemia and its peripheral effects; excessive production of adrenal androgens induce hypertrichosis, hirsutism, and clitoromegaly. Increased levels of androgens early in life induce formation of ambiguous external genitals such as may be found in congenital adrenal hyperplasia. These ambiguous changes are not seen in acquired or postpubertal forms of adrenal androgen excess. Conversion of the androgens to 17β-estradiol, as well as an increased production of this estrogen by the hyperplastic adrenal, disturb regulation of the hypothalamic-pituitary-gonadal axis, with resulting amenorrhea. Disturbed menstrual cyclicity in idiopathic adrenocortical insufficiency may be due to associated autoimmune disturbance of the gonads, but, in tuberculous adrenal insufficiency, it is a reflection of hypogonadotropinism secondary to inanition. In adrenal insufficiency, the clinical stigmata also include hypotension, weakness, hyperpigmentation, and hypoglycemia. Similar clinical features relative to the reproductive tract are found in biosynthetic adrenal defects in which excessive amounts of androgens are produced. These include defects in 21-hydroxylase, in 11β-hydroxylase, and hydroxysteroid dehydrogenase. In these disorders, there are no stigmata of hypercortisolemia. Clinical descriptions of these disorders are presented in detail in Chapter 10. Adrenocortical hyperplasia with 21-hydroxylase deficiency in the congenital form is associated with ambiguous genitals, and, if persistent, with clitoromegaly, hirsutism, and occasional problems of sexual identity. Acquired, postpubertal forms are characterized by virilization and amenorrhea. A congenital defect in adrenal 11β-hydroxylase is characterized by ambiguous genitals, other evidence of virilization, hypokalemic alkalosis and hypertension, and eventual amenorrhea. In the postpubertal form, the major manifestations include virilization, amenorrhea, and hypertension with hypokalemic alkalosis. Hydroxysteroid dehydrogenase deficiency in the congenital form is a basis of ambiguous genitals and may later be manifested by virilization and amenorrhea. In a rare form of adrenocortical hyperplasia associated with a biosynthetic defect, a deficiency of the enzyme 17α-hydroxylase occurs in both the adrenals and the gonads. Because this step is essential in the production of both androgens and estrogens, the major clinical manifestations include sexual infantilism (hypogonadism). Associated clinical effects are hypertension and hypokalemic alkalosis secondary to hypermineralocorticoidism.

Evaluation of patients with amenorrhea for possible adrenocortical defects will, therefore, depend on the clinical manifestations. The patient with virilization, ambiguous genitals, hirsutism, and clitoromegaly should be studied for increased levels of testosterone or other androgens. In both the 21-hydroxylase and 11β-hydroxylase defects, the androgenic substance is mainly testosterone. In these disorders, there are also elevated levels of urinary pregnanatriol, derived from 17-hydroxyprogesterone, which accumulates in the 21-hydroxylase defect; and in tetrahydrodesoxycortisol (THS) which accumulates in the 11β-hydroxylase defect. The active androgen in the hydroxysteroid defect is dehydroepiandrosterone, which may be quantitated as such or as 17-KS in the urine. Urinary 17-KS are also elevated whenever there is an increase in androstenedione which may occur in the 21-hydroxylase and 11β-hydroxylase deficiencies. Deficiency of the 17α-hydroxylase is confirmed by decreased levels of 17-KS, estrogens, and increased levels of C 21-compounds of the non-17-hydroxylated series, i.e., 11-desoxycorticosterone (DOC), corticosterone (B), and their respective reduction products, THDOC and THB.

Depending on the type of defect, elevated levels of the specific hormones or metabolites listed above or of 17-KS and 17-ketogenic steroids, may be further evaluated by determining if the elevated levels are suppressible by administration of exogenous corticosteroids, e.g., prednisone, dexamethasone, or cortisol. Suppressibility is evidence that ACTH excess, secondary to a decreased cortisol produced by the adrenal, is present. Nonsuppressibility would be indicative of an autonomous process, as in adrenocortical neoplasm.

Suppression of the urine or plasma levels of the steroid metabolites with an exogenous corticosteroid has been employed quite extensively to determine the presence of adrenal hyperplasia associated with a biosynthetic defect. Despite the logic that such suppressibility reflects ACTH-dependence, and its widespread usefulness, the reliability of this procedure is being questions (Kirschner and Bardin, 1972).

To perform the test, baseline levels of urinary 17-KS, 17-KGS, 17-OHCS, pregnanetriol, or THS and plasma testosterone are obtained. The patient is then given 0.5 mg of dexamethasone 4 times daily for 3 days. The urine for the above measurements is collected on the last day of steroid ingestion. Plasma testosterone is drawn on the morning after completion of the dexamethasone dosage. Suppression of any of these parameters is good evidence of ACTH dependence and, therefore, of adrenal hyperplasia. Nonsuppression would suggest an autonomous adrenal problem as a neoplasm, or a non-adrenal source, of the metabolites. It should be clear that pregnantriol, THS, and 17-KGS would be clearly indicative of an adrenal source. It is not necessary to measure all of the metabolites listed above since clinical judgment should prompt the direction of the search. For example, the presence of virilization without hypertension, obesity, or carbohydrate intolerance should prompt examination of metabolites expected in 21-hydroxylase deficiency. Similarly, the presence of hypertension, hypokalemic alkalosis, and virilization should prompt pursuit of 11β-hydroxylase deficiency, and, therefore, of assessment of 17-KS and THS, as well as testosterone. It is recommended that, if plasma testosterone is employed as the parameter before and after dexamethasone challenge, plasma cortisol levels should also be determined. A suppression of cortisol without an accompanying testosterone decrease would indicate that the adrenal process is under ACTH control whereas the source of testosterone is not. Nonsuppressibility of both would suggest an extra-adrenal source or an autonomous adrenal tumor.

The dexamethasone plus human chorionic gonadotropin (HCG) challenge has also been employed extensively to determine responsiveness of the ovaries to gonadotropic stimulation. The test is performed as follows: one or two 24-hr urine samples are obtained for 17-KS determinations, and a baseline plasma testosterone level is determined. The patient is then given 0.5–0.75 mg of dexamethasone 4 times daily for 7–10 days to achieve complete suppression of the pituitary-adrenal axis. At the end of 7 days, urinary 17-KS and plasma testosterone are again determined. While the patient continues to receive dexamethasone, she is given 4,000 units of HCG intramuscularly daily for 3 doses. On the day of the last injection, the above parameters are again monitored. Significant increases in plasma testosterone and urinary 17-KS after the HCG stimulation would suggest the ovaries as the source of the increases. Such changes are observed in patients with polycystic ovarian disease, but not in normal women.

The suppressibility of elevated testosterone by procedures which suppress ovarian activity is employed to determine the origin of the androgen. The most widely employed test utilizing this concept is the dexamethasone-

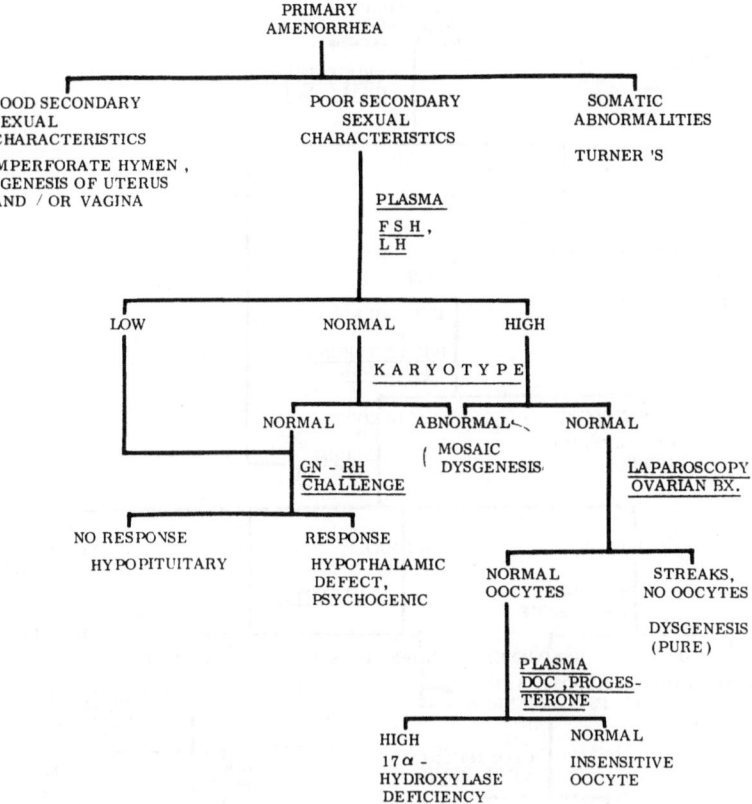

Figure 6.3. Diagram for diagnosis of primary amenorrhea utilizing clinical findings and various hormone measurements as well as physiologic manipulations to determine autonomy of the involved steroid-secreting glands. See figure 6.4.

diethyl stilbestrol test. In this procedure, the adrenal cortex is suppressed by dexamethasone as above. The patient is then given 5 mg of diethylstilbestrol twice daily for 10 days. Suppression of an elevated testosterone by diethylstilbestrol in the absence of suppression by dexamethasone is good evidence that the androgen is derived from an ovarian source which is under gonadotropin control. These procedures are employed in the flow sheets for diagnosis of amenorrhea in figures 6.3 and 6.4. Additional procedures are described in Chapter 10.

Amenorrhea Secondary to Diseases of the Thyroid

As described previously, menstrual cyclicity is affected by disorders of thyroid function either by direct effect on the hypothalamic nuclei or on the turnover of estrogens, thus affecting the feedback regulation of gonadotropin secretion. Thyroid function tests are discussed in detail in another section,

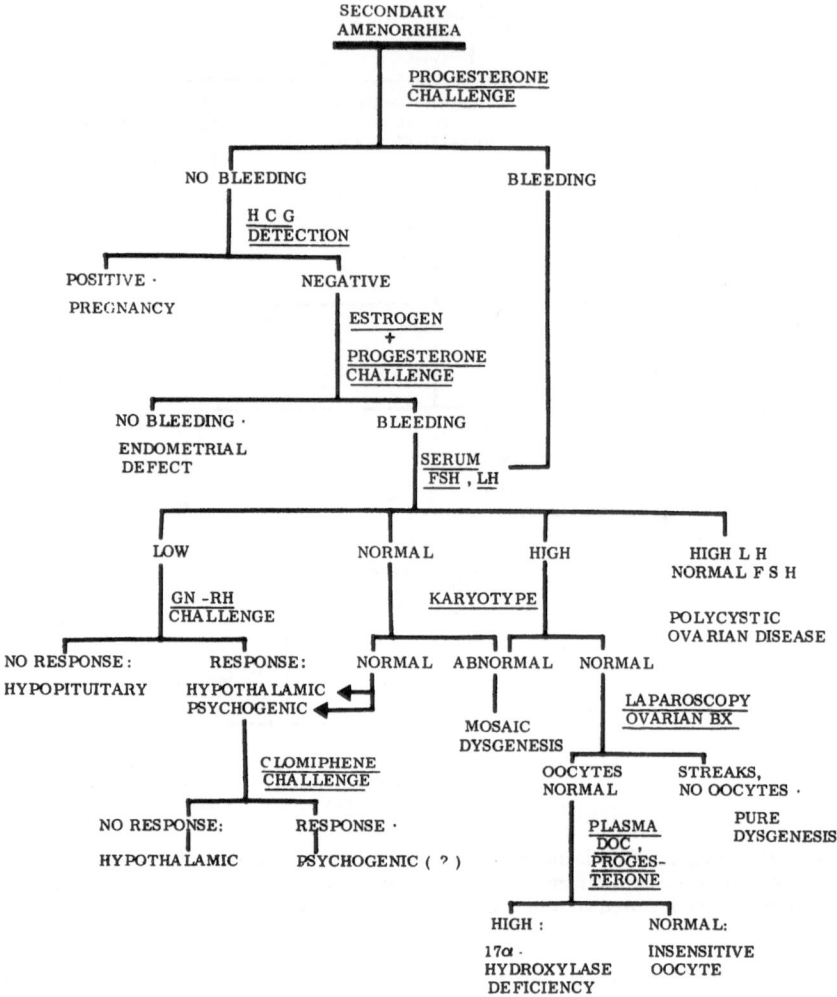

Figure 6.4. Diagram for diagnosis of secondary amenorrhea. See explanation to figure 6.3.

but the most reliable tests to evaluate functions of this gland will be summarized here. For confirmation of the diagnosis of hypothyroidism, the following panel is most reliable; serum thyroxin level (by RIA); resin uptake of T_3 (or other method of TBG assessment); and serum TSH. The TBG assessment permits correction of the total T_4 value for the amount of TBG. To evaluate the etiology of the hypothyroidism requires additional clinical and laboratory data as indicated in another section. Hyperthyroidism is best authenticated by serum levels of T_4 corrected by an assessment of TBG and by the serum levels of T_3 (by RIA). Establishment of the etiology of hyperthyroidism requires additional clinical and laboratory information as outlined in Chapter 9.

Evaluation of amenorrhea due to other systemic disorders requires a complete history and physical examination as well as a broad-based approach to determine the presence of occult or overt systemic illnesses. Such procedures should include a chest X-ray, a skull X-ray, complete hemogram, erythrocyte sedimentation rate, serum electrolytes, serum albumin and globulins, blood glucose, serum alkaline phosphatase, serum glutamic oxaloacetic transaminase, lactate dehydrogenase, blood urea nitrogen and creatinine, urinalysis, and electrocardiogram. Findings from the above screening procedures should prompt definitive workup of any single abnormal finding or combination of abnormal findings.

MANAGEMENT OF AMENORRHEA

Management of amenorrheic syndromes requires cognizance of the pathophysiologic basis of the disorder. It is essential to assure the patient that the lack of menstruation *per se* does not represent a threat to life expectancy. It is equally important for the physician to establish whether the amenorrhea represents a manifestation of a chronic disabling or life-threatening disease. If such serious disorders are ruled out by appropriate clinical and laboratory studies, then due consideration is given to the need of estrogen therapy for prevention of clinical effects of such deficiency. Artificial cycles should not be induced unless appropriate studies eliminate serious underlying disorders as basis for amenorrhea.

In patients with cryptomenorrhea, there is no need for hormonal therapy. Appropriate surgical and mechanical procedures should be employed to ensure patency of the cervical and vaginal tracts. In patients with uterine agenesis and probable endometrial nonresponsiveness, definitive treatment is virtually nonexistent. Plastic surgical procedures may be helpful in patients with vaginal agenesis.

Treatment of patients with hypergonadotropic hypogonadism depends on the nature of the disturbance. Those with gonadal dysgenesis should be given cyclic hormone therapy. Several forms of hormone replacement are available, but the recommended regimens require the administration of diethylstilbesterol (0.5 mg daily) or premarin (1.25 mg daily) for 20 days each month. Progestational agent in the form of 5 mg of medroxyprogesterone is given daily for the last 5 days of estrogen therapy to provide secretory changes in the endometrium and eventual sloughing on withdrawal of the hormones. It is important to recognize that use of the oral contraceptive agents for the above purposes is not recommended as these preparations contain pharmacologic amounts of the hormones.

A most common form of physiologic hypergonadotropic hypogonadism is the menopause. Atrophic changes in the ovaries preclude any follicular response to the gonadotropins with resultant anovulation and decreased levels of estrogens. Several acute clinical manifestations, including vasomotor symptoms and hot flashes, referable to this change in levels of estrogens, occur in menopausal women. Chronic sequelae ascribed to hypoestrogenism include osteoporosis, atherosclerosis, and atrophic changes in the vaginal tract. The management of patients who exhibit the acute effects of estrogen deficiency entails psychologic support as well as replacement dosages of estrogens. Despite previous opinions that the hot flashes were ascribable to hypergonadotropinism, the occurrence of these acute vasomotor symptoms after removal of the pituitary negates this explanation. It is quite likely that the most severe acute manifestations of hypoestrogenism, including hot flashes and emotional disturbances, occur in women who were neurotic or prepsychotic premenopausally. Some patients also develop hypertension, arthralgias, and diabetes mellitus, but the pathogenetic relationship of hypoestrogenism to these manifestations is not clear.

Many of the acute manifestations of the menopause are controlled by estrogen replacement. It is likely that the required dosages may be lower than required to suppress the increased levels of FSH and LH, but this has not been definitively proved. The possible usefulness of plasma determinations of FSH and LH to determine the minimal effective doses of estrogens should be considered.

A recommended regimen consists of oral doses of 0.02 mg of estinyl estradiol, or 0.625–1.25 mg of congugated estrogen (Premarin daily for 3 out of 4 wk). There are no definitive data to indicate any superiority of parenteral estrogens in this disorder. The doses of estrogens recommended are probably quite safe in regard to their possible oncogenetic potential, but it is advisable nevertheless that these patients should be followed up at intervals, at which time periodic physical examinations are conducted.

Osteoporosis and atherosclerosis frequently accompany menopause and are especially significant in patients with premature menopause (spontaneous or postsurgical). It is likely that these processes are irreversible once they begin. Early estrogen replacement should be instituted in the younger patients, but should probably be seriously considered in all menopausal patients if there are no overt contraindications. Objective criteria for the appropriate dosages and duration of therapy are lacking. The possible usefulness of monitoring plasma FSH as an index of estrogen replacement has not been fully tested. The probable insensitivity of the hypothalamic nuclei to estrogens in older patients with the menopause may be an argument against this index. FSH monitoring may be more helpful in patients with premature menopause.

Estrogen replacement may cause an abatement in bone resorption in menopause, but this is of limited duration. Androgen therapy has proved essentially ineffective in this regard also.

Recent studies suggest possible reversal of bone destruction by instituting a therapeutic regimen of calcium replacement (as Neocalglucon, 325 mg 2 or 3 times daily; vitamin D, 50,000 units twice weekly; and sodium fluoride, 40 mg daily). The patient is advised to indulge in regular physical activities while on this regimen.

Several methods for management of polycystic ovarian disease (Stein-Leventhal syndrome) have been tried, and none with complete satisfaction, perhaps owing to the probability that the disease mechanisms may differ in patients. Wedge resection of the ovaries has often been followed by re-establishment of menstrual cycles and pregnancy. Most patients revert to the pattern of amenorrhea or oligomenorrhea after several months. The signs of virilization and hypertrichosis are not altered by the surgery. Several studies have shown that approximately 30–40% of patients with this disorder may improve with dexamethasone (0.5–0.75 mg daily) or prednisone (2.5–5 mg daily) suppression of the pituitary-adrenal axis. During a period of therapy, these patients have regular menses, ovulate, have become pregnant, and some (around 30%) have had decrease or disappearance of hirsutism. It is likely that this group has major adrenocortical component in the disorder. Many patients with proven Stein-Leventhal syndrome have been stimulated to ovulation and eventual pregnancy. The management involves the use of clomiphene citrate which is given as follows. The patient is given 50 mg of clomiphene orally daily for 5 days starting on the fifth day of the cycle, with an increase up to 150 mg daily for 5 days in subsequent cycles. Patients who fail to ovulate to clomiphene stimulation are treated with HCG (10,000 units intramuscularly 2 days after the last clomiphene dose). Patients are tried on this regimen for 6 months, and if ovulation is not induced, then the alternative methods of treatment may be tried. This regimen fails to alter the pattern of hirsutism.

Patients with the Stein-Leventhal syndrome who do not desire fertility may be treated with cyclic estrogen-progesterone therapy. Some of these may have remarkable improvement in the hirsutism.

Management of hypoestrogenism and amenorrhea secondary to decreased or absent levels of FSH and LH requires knowledge of the underlying mechanism of the defect in release of the hormones. Treatable life-threatening intracranial problems should be treated appropriately. Vascular anomalies, if correctible, and infectious diseases are managed by the appropriate methods. Restitution of ovulation and menses are required mainly for purposes of childbearing; otherwise, hormonal therapy is restricted to prevention of chronic effects of hypoestrogenism. Regimens simulating the normal release of FSH and LH have resulted in ovulation and successful pregnancies in several patients. One standard regimen employs human pituitary extract rich in FSH (HPFSH) 250–500 units daily for 10 days, followed by 3,000–6,000

IU of HCG daily for 3 days, in management of infertility. This regimen resulted in pregnancies in more than 43%, of whom 44% had multiple births and 26% ended in abortion. Ovarian hyperstimulation and ascites were seen in some patients. Lack of sufficient supply of HPFSH precludes its underspread usage in these disorders.

An extract of human menopausal urine with high FSH activity (Pergonal) has been employed in combination with HCG in the management of infertility due to anovulation. The patient is given a 12-day course of therapy with Pergonal followed by 3 days of HCG. The induction of ovulation and subsequent pregnancy by this regimen is established. Multiple births and abortions were also noted in some of the treated patients.

Both methods of gonadotropin therapy may precipitate the ovarian hyperstimulation syndrome, consisting of abdominal pain, bloating, pressure, nausea, and malaise. Ovarian rupture and hemorrhage have also been observed after this regimen.

Despite the presence of an otherwise intact hypothalamic-pituitary-ovarian system, amenorrhea may result from disturbances in the feedback regulation of this axis. Hepatic disease, nutritional problems, starvation, diabetes mellitus, and thyroid dysfunction may affect hypothalamic function by altering the degradation of estradiol. Decreases in release, and probably synthesis, of pituitary hormones have been observed in starvation and dietary deficiency states, and correctible by realimentation. Disturbed feedback regulation of the axis may also be seen in disorders of the adrenal cortex in which overproduction of estrogens or increased peripheral conversion of androgen to estradiol may be present. Definitive management of these errors in regulation of the hypothalamic-pituitary-ovarian axis are described in the appropriate chapters.

MANAGEMENT OF HIRSUTISM

Hirsutism is a feature of many of the disorders of menstrual cycles and infertility discussed above and in Chapters 5 and 10. Because this finding is a reflection of excessive androgen action, the recognized etiologies are related to androgen production by the ovaries, the adrenals, or androgen-producing ovarian neoplasms (Chapter 10). The syndrome in idiopathic hirsutism is presumed to be due to androgen overproduction by the adrenal cortex. Pathogenesis of the Stein-Leventhal syndrome is not clear, but ovarian and/or adrenal androgen production may be responsible for hirsutism found in several patients with this disorder. It is becoming clear that, in several patients with unexplained hirsutism, there is an end-organ hyperresponsiveness to normal amounts of androgens. The participation of sex hormone-binding globulin and competition between androgens and estrogens for this binding substance should be considered in the pathogenetic mechanism. The possible increased avidity of cytosol steroid receptor in appropriate target organs may also be relevant in this regard.

Establishment of the source of the androgen in hirsutism states involves measurements of urinary 17-ketosteroids and plasma testosterone, androstenedione, and dehydroepiandrosterone. In most patients with hirsutism, there are high levels of androstenedione. Appropriate suppression and stimulation tests are employed to determine the source of the androgens. Recent data suggest that dexamethasone suppressibility is not necessarily diagnostic of an adrenocortical source (Kirschner and Bardin, 1972) of the androgens. Several of the physiologic manipulations employed in the differential diagnosis of amenorrhea associated with virilization are employed in the study of hirsutism.

In patients with hirsutism in whom the basis is identified, *e.g.*, Cushing's syndrome or masculinizing ovarian tumors, successful surgical therapy is followed by (resolution of the excessive hair growth in most patients. Hirsutism due to virilizing adrenocortical hyperplasia improves in about 35–50% of the patients after several months of dexamethasone suppression therapy. Hirsutism associated with the Stein-Leventhal syndrome rarely improves after wedge resection despite permanent or temporary restitution of menstrual cyclicity. Patients with the Stein-Leventhal syndrome and with idiopathic hirsutism may reveal patterns of suppressibility of previously elevated plasma testosterone after dexamethasone challenge, and their hirsutism may respond to continued dexamethasone suppression. A regimen of 0.5 mg of dexamethasone daily along with a high estrogen oral contraceptive has resulted in decreased hair growth in 40–50% of patients under our care.

REFERENCES

Abraham, G. E., J. R. Marshall, et al. 1972. Disorders of Ovulation. *In* N. D. Assali (ed.), Pathology of Gestation. Academic Press, Inc., New York.

Ansari, A. H., and R. Cowdrey. 1974. Gravlee Jet Washer for endometrial dating. Fertil. & Steril. 25:127–144.

Bacchus, H. 1968. Clinical laboratory procedures for determination of urinary 17-hydroxy-21-deoxycorticosteroids. Am. J. Clin. Path. 59:351–359.

Bacchus, H. 1972. Endocrine profiles in the clinical laboratory. *In* M. Stefanini (ed.), Progress in Clinical Pathology. Vol. 4. Grune & Stratton, Inc., New York. pp 1–101.

Gambrell, R. D., R. B. Greenblatt, and V. B. Mahesh. 1973. Inappropriate secretion of LH in the Stein-Leventhal syndrome. Obst. & Gynec. 42:429–440.

Harsoulis, P., J. C. Marshall, S. F. Kuku, C. W. Burke, D. K. London, and T.

R. Fraser. 1974. Combined test for assessment of anterior pituitary function. Brit. Med. J. 4:326–329.

Hertz, R., W. D. Odell, et al. 1966. Diagnostic implications of primary amenorrhea. Am. Int. Med. 65:800–820.

Kirschner, M. A., and C. W. Bardin. 1972. Androgen production and metabolism in normal and virilized women. Metabolism 21:667–688.

Kirschner, M. A., J. R. Zucker, and D. Jespersen. 1974. Adult adrenogenital syndrome. Does it exist? Abstract #6, Proceedings of Meeting of American College of Physicians, New York.

Lipssett, M. D., and M. A. Kirschner. 1970. Malignant lipid cell tumor of the ovary: Clinical, biochemical and etiological considerations. J. Clin. Endocrinol. 30:336–344.

Lloyd, C. W., J. Lobotsky, et al. 1966. Plasma testosterone and urinary 17-KS in women with hirsutism and polycystic ovaries. J. Clin. Endocrinol. 26: 314–322.

Philip, J., V. Sele and. 1965. Primary amenorrhea. A study of 101 cases. Fertil. & Steril. 16:795.

Prunty, F. T. G., and R. V. Brooks. 1960. Patterns of steroid excretion in three types of post-puberal hirsutism. J. Endocrinol. 21: 263–275.

Stein, J. F., and Leventhal, M. L. 1935. Amenorrhea associated with bilateral polycystic ovaries. Am. J. Obstet. & Gynecol. 29:181–191.

Taymor, M. L., and R. Barnard. 1962. Luteinizing hormone excretion in the polycystic ovary syndrome. Fertil. & Steril. 13:510–512.

Yen, S. S. C., P. Vela, and. 1970. Inappropriate secretion of FSH and LH in polycystic ovarian disease. J. Clin. Endocrinol. 30:435–442.

Zarate, A., A. J. Kastin, J. Soria, et al. 1973. Effect of synthetic luteinizing hormone release hormone (LH-RH) in two brothers with hypogonadism and anosmia. J. Clin. Endocrinol. 36:612–614.

Zarate, A., J. Soria, E. S. Canales, et al. 1973. Pituitary FSH and LH reserve in women with isolated gonadotropin deficiency. Obst. & Gynecol. 42:507–510.

7
Infertility

Infertility is defined as failure to achieve conception during one or more years of intercourse without use of any contraceptive measure (Behrman and Kistner, 1968). Primary infertility refers to the lack of pregnancy as defined above. Secondary infertility occurs in patients who were previously pregnant but fail to conceive during one or more years of unprotected intercourse. It is estimated that 10–15% of couples in the United States are infertile. Absolute infertility refers to totally irremediable bases of the problem, whereas relative infertility occurs in conditions which are correctible after diagnosis. Several factors may be responsible for the occurrence of infertility, including problems in the male as well as female components of the marital unit. In both sexes there are genetic-endocrine-metabolic, as well as mechanical factors, as the basis.

MALE INFERTILITY

In males, the genetic-endocrine-metabolic factors include various defects in the process in spermatogenesis, as occur in congenital problems such as cryptorchidism, Klinefelter's syndrome, postpubertal panhypopituitarism, and seminiferous tubule failure. Mechanical defects include ductal obstruction, spontaneous or induced. Other factors ascribable to the male component include infrequent intercourse, poor timing, and immunologic incompatibility.

Analysis of the male component includes medical history and physical examination, sperm count, and, when appropriate, studies on testosterone, FSH and LH, and testicular biopsy. Table 7.1 presents clinical laboratory data on male hypogonadal syndromes. Of the disorders listed, most of the hypergonadotropic hypogonadal syndromes are associated with azoospermia and, therefore, with infertility. Exceptions in this grouping include some forms of adult Leydig cell failure in which sperm counts are normal. Among the forms of hypogonadotropic hypogonadism, the "fertile eunuch" syndrome is capa-

Table 7.1. Laboratory Diagnosis of Male Hypogonadal Syndromes[a]

Disorder[b]	Clinical features	Sperm count	Plasma or urine		
			Testosterone	FSH	LH
Hypergonadotropic					
Klinefelter's	Gynecomastia; small testis	0	Low normal	High	High
Reifenstein's	Hypospadias; gynecomastia	0	Low	High	High
Functional prepubertal castrate	Short stature; empty scrotum	0	Low	High	High
Male Turner's	Mental retardation, cryptorchidism; gynecomastia; short stature	0	Low	High	High
Sertoli-cell-only syndrome	Gynecomastia absent	0	Normal	High	Normal
Adult seminiferous tubule failure; mumps orchitis, idiopathic, or in myotonic dystrophy	Normal development; no overt physical findings, except in myotonic dystrophy where there are myotonia, baldness, and lens defects	Decreased or absent	Normal (low in mumps orchitis)	High	Normal (high in mumps orchitis)
Adult Leydig cell failure	Hot flashes, decreased libido	Normal	Normal or low	High	High

Hypogonadotropic
Hypogonadotropic eunuchoidism

Complete or typical (Kallman's)	Eunuchoid features; small testes; anosmia or hyposmia	0	Low	Low	Low
Incomplete	Cleft palate; craniofacial dyssymmetry	0 or low	Low	Low or normal	Low or normal
Delayed puberty	Slow maturation only	0 or low	Low	Low or normal	Low or normal
Fertile eunuch	Eunuchoidal	Low	Low	Low to normal	Low or normal
Prepubertal panhypopituitarism	Lack of growth; sexual infantilism	0 or low	Low	Low	Low
Postpubertal pituitary failure (panhypopituitarism)	Decreased libido; impotence; regression of secondary sex characteristics	0 or low	Low	Low to normal	Low to normal

[a]Extragonadal causes of hypogonadism include myxedema, Cushing's syndrome, and adrenal insufficiency.

[b]Chromatin pattern or buccal smear is negative in all except occasionally in Klinefelter's syndrome, where it may be negative. The chromosome karyotype is XY in all except in Klinefelter's, where it may be XXY, poly X + Y, or mosaic; and in male Turner's syndrome, where it may be XY or poly X + Y.

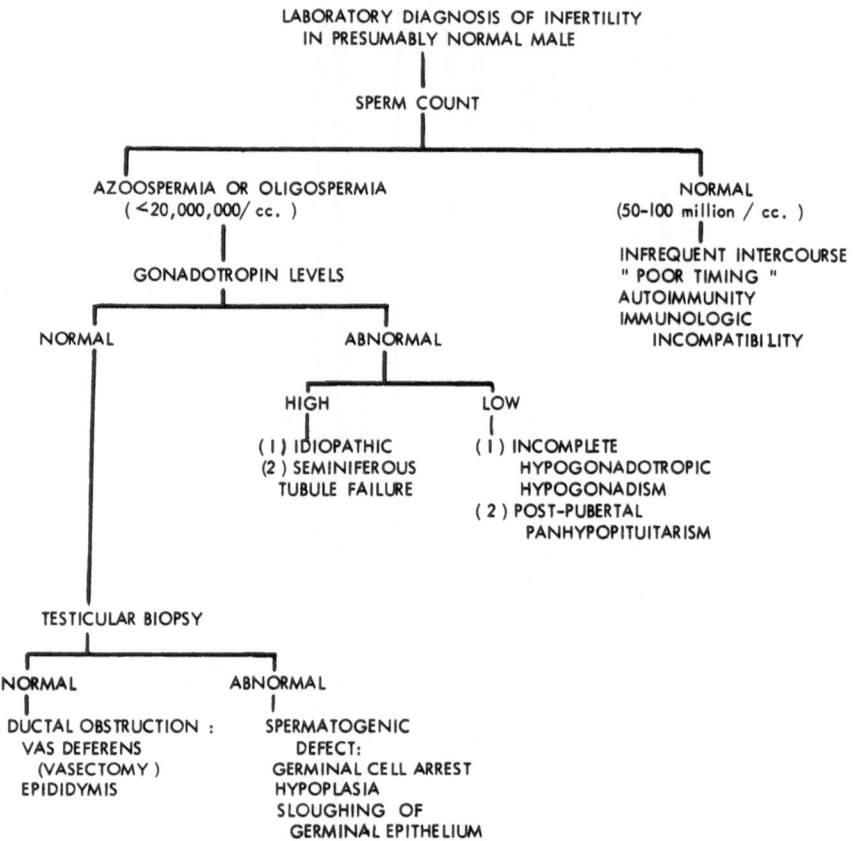

LABORATORY DIAGNOSIS OF INFERTILITY
IN PRESUMABLY NORMAL MALE

SPERM COUNT

AZOOSPERMIA OR OLIGOSPERMIA
(<20,000,000/ cc.)

NORMAL
(50-100 million / cc.)

INFREQUENT INTERCOURSE
" POOR TIMING "
AUTOIMMUNITY
IMMUNOLOGIC
INCOMPATIBILITY

GONADOTROPIN LEVELS

NORMAL

ABNORMAL

HIGH

(I) IDIOPATHIC
(2) SEMINIFEROUS
TUBULE FAILURE

LOW

(I) INCOMPLETE
HYPOGONADOTROPIC
HYPOGONADISM
(2) POST-PUBERTAL
PANHYPOPITUITARISM

TESTICULAR BIOPSY

NORMAL

DUCTAL OBSTRUCTION :
VAS DEFERENS
(VASECTOMY)
EPIDIDYMIS

ABNORMAL

SPERMATOGENIC
DEFECT:
GERMINAL CELL ARREST
HYPOPLASIA
SLOUGHING OF
GERMINAL EPITHELIUM

Figure 7.1. Diagram for laboratory diagnosis of male infertility.

ble of significant spermatogenesis. Diagnostic workup of infertility in the male is presented in the flow diagram in figure 7.1 (Bacchus, 1972).

FEMALE INFERTILITY

In addition to viable spermatozoa from the male, fertilization and implantation in the female require the processes of ovulation, production of cervical mucus appropriate for support and transport of the spermatozoa, tubal patency, and the availability of an adequate endometrial implantation site. Mechanical factors which inhibit these processes include: (1) defects in tubal patency and peristaltic activity; (2) uterine leiomyomata; (3) endometriosis; (4) infectious disorders, such as gonorrhea or tuberculosis; (5) chronic pelvic inflammation leading to tubal occlusion and chronic endocervicitis; (6) malpositions or congenital malformations of the uterus; and (7) cervical incompetence. Clinical features of the above disorders are summarized in table 7.2. Endocrine factors responsible for infertility in the female include errors in the menstrual cycle such as: (1) dysfunctional uterine bleeding (or dysfunctional metrorrhagia), in which the follicular phase and estrogen production are intact, but ovulation and luteinization usually do not occur, and the growing follicle forms a retention cyst; and (2) amenorrhea, in which both the follicular and corpus luteal phases are affected. In all disturbances of the menstrual cycle, the possible defects in operation of the hypothalamic-pituitary-ovarian axis must be considered. The most common cause of amenorrhea associated with infertility is a functional disturbance of this axis. Such disturbance may reside at the level of the hypothalamus, the pituitary, or the gonads, as well as in the feedback control of the axis by levels of ovarian hormones. Ambient levels of these hormones are influenced not only by production rates, but also by the rate of breakdown and conversion. These processes are influenced by various factors, such as activities of the thyroid and adrenals, nutritional and disease history, and drug effects. It is also essential that evidence is obtained on the responsiveness of the endometrium to hormonal stimulation and withdrawal. The various endocrinologic causes of infertility are listed in figure 7.2 according to the location of the defect along the hypothalamic to ovarian axis. These disorders have been considered in Chapters 6, 9, and 10. The clinical features of these disorders are presented in summary form in table 7.2.

Evaluation of Infertility in the Female Patient

Union of the sperm and ovum in the ampulla of the oviduct is dependent on the anatomic and functional integrity of the female reproductive tract. It is, therefore, essential that the competence of this tract is investigated in cases of female infertility (Bacchus, 1972; Israel, 1967). Considerations on the work-up of male infertility were considered previously.

Competence of the Fallopian tubes is evaluated by: (1) the Rubin test, which involves tubal insufflation with carbon dioxide; (2) hysterosalpingography, which is a radiologic method of evaluation patency of the tract; and (3) direct visualization by culdoscopy or laparoscopy.

(1) The Rubin test requires a transcervical introduction of carbon dioxide under carefully controlled pressure and flow rate. The gas progresses through the uterus and the ostia of the tubes, and finally into the peritoneal cavity. The occurrence of referred shoulder pain and X-ray appearance of air under the diaphragm constitute a positive test indicating patency of the tubal system. If such findings do not occur under gas pressure of 200 mm of Hg, then the test is discontinued and is considered indicative of tubal incompetence. Because the negative test may occasionally result from tubal spasm, it

Table 7.2. Infertility in the Female

Disorder	Nature of defect	Clinical manifestation	Key laboratory data
Hypopituitarism	Defect in FSH and LH release; generalized endocrine abnormality	Insidious onset; slowly progressive disorder with clinical manifestations of loss of GH, thyroid hormones, cortisol, and gonadal hormones[a]	Plasma FSH and LH, TSH, ACTH, GH, cortisol low and nonresponsive appropriate stimulation challenges
Thyroid diseases	Disturbances in estradiol feedback to hypothalamus; also generalized endocrine disturbance	Chronic disorder; insidious onset; manifestations of hypothyroidism or hyperthyroidism; fertility often restored with treatment[b]	Hypothyroidism Low T_4, RUT_3, and RAI uptake; high TSH Hyperthyroidism Elevated T_4, T_3, RUT and RAI uptake
Adrenal disease Cushing's syndrome	Generalized endocrine disturbance	Errors in menstrual cyclicity; hypertension; centripetal fat distribution; hirsutism, osteoporosis	High plasma cortisol without circadian cyclicity; nonsuppressible with dethamethasone, urine 17-OHCS, 17-KGS and 17-KS elevated
Biosynthetic defects	Disturbed feedback control of FSH and LH	Hirsutism; amenorrhea (in C 21 hydroxylase deficiency); hypertension and hypokalemic alkalosis (in 11β-hydroxylase deficiency); sexual infantilism, hypertension, and hypokalemic alkalosis (in 17α-hydroxylase deficiency)[c]	Elevated THS and THDOC (in 11β-hydroxylase deficiency); elevated THB and THDOC (in 17α-hydroxylase deficiency); elevated 17-KS (in all except 17α-hydroxylase deficiency)

Stein-Leventhal syndrome	Disturbance in pituitary control of ovary (?); inappropriate LH elevation; increased androgens	Gradual onset irregular menses to amenorrhea; hirsutism in many; ovaries with characteristic appearance; fertility often restored after therapy[d]	Elevated testosterone; increased LH and normal FSH; culdoscopy or laparoscopy reveal characteristic ovaries
Turner's syndrome	Chromosomal induced anomaly in gonadal development; XO, XX, XX[b] variants	Congenital and permanent infertility; primary amenorrhea; characteristic somatic findings[d]	Chromatin negative; abnormal karyotype; low estradiol, increased FSH and LH
Cervicitis, vaginitis, and gonorrhea	Infection or trauma	Evidence of inflammatory response; tubal potency affected; fertility restored with treatment	Gross appearance and microbiologic finding
Uterine tumors; endometriosis	Mechanical defects	Dysmenorrhea; menorrhagia, nodular uterus, other physical findings	Culdoscopy or laparoscopy pelvic examination

[a] See Chapters 3, 6, 9, and 10.
[b] See Chapter 9.
[c] See Chapter 10.
[d] See Chapter 6.

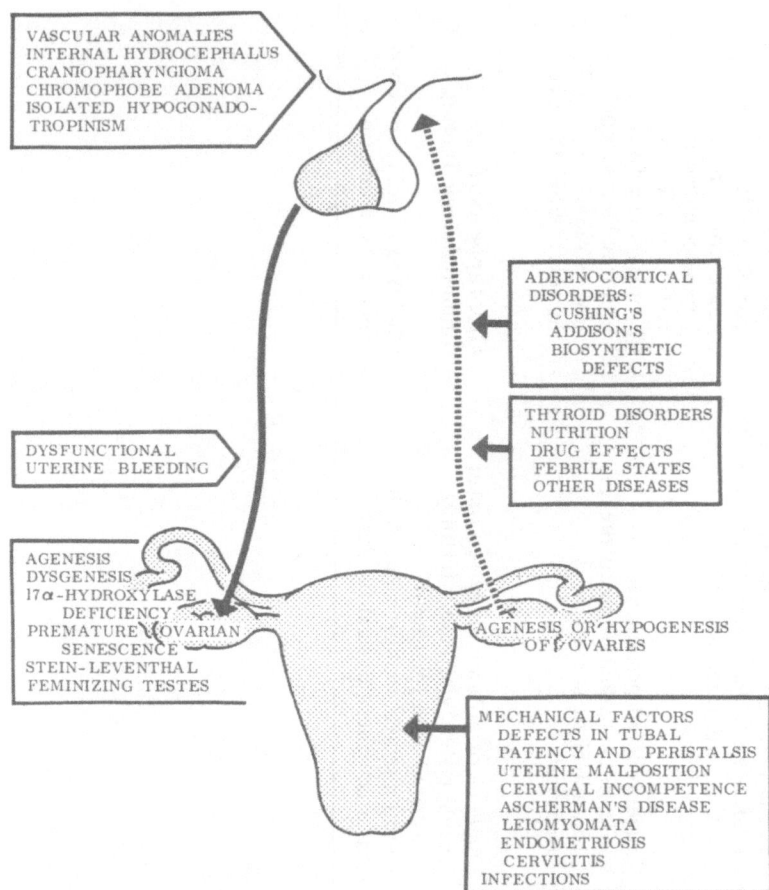

VASCULAR ANOMALIES
INTERNAL HYDROCEPHALUS
CRANIOPHARYNGIOMA
CHROMOPHOBE ADENOMA
ISOLATED HYPOGONADO-
TROPINISM

ADRENOCORTICAL
DISORDERS:
   CUSHING'S
   ADDISON'S
   BIOSYNTHETIC
      DEFECTS

THYROID DISORDERS
NUTRITION
DRUG EFFECTS
FEBRILE STATES
OTHER DISEASES

DYSFUNCTIONAL
UTERINE BLEEDING

AGENESIS
DYSGENESIS
17α-HYDROXYLASE
   DEFICIENCY
PREMATURE OVARIAN
   SENESCENCE
STEIN-LEVENTHAL
FEMINIZING TESTES

AGENESIS OR HYPOGENESIS
   OF OVARIES

MECHANICAL FACTORS
DEFECTS IN TUBAL
PATENCY AND PERISTALSIS
UTERINE MALPOSITION
CERVICAL INCOMPETENCE
ASCHERMAN'S DISEASE
LEIOMYOMATA
ENDOMETRIOSIS
CERVICITIS
INFECTIONS

Figure 7.2. Etiologies of female infertility presented against the hypothalamic-pituitary-ovarian axis and feedback circuit. See explanation to figure 6.1.

is advisable that the procedure be repeated under paracervical block local anesthesia. Continued infertility despite a positive Rubin test may necessitate additional studies to rule out tubal distortion or adhesions.

(2) Hysterosalpingography involves the instillation of 3–6 cc of a radio-opaque oil into the uterine cavity and oviducts under fluoroscopic guidance. Distribution of the dye is determined by X-rays taken at the time of instillation and 24 hr later. Obstructive phenomena are readily recorded by this procedure.

(3) Culdoscopy, combined with tubal insufflation with methylene blue, provides a very effective method of detecting adhesions and other obstructive phenomena. Laparoscopy permits visual evidence of these processes also.

An extremely useful test which provides information on the adequacy of coital position, intromission, ejaculate content and quality, or cervical environment is the postcoital test. The test is performed at the expected time of ovulation, at not less than 2 hr or more than 16 hr after intercourse. Best data are obtained at 4–6 hr after intercourse, following a few days of sexual intercourse. Specimens of endocervical and vaginal mucus are examined for clarity, ferning pattern, elasticity, and the number and motility of the spermatozoa. Best sperm survival occurs in clear, abundant, and elastic mucus. (It is essential that the sperm count and motility studies in this test not be considered substitute for definitive studies in the male partner.) Unsatisfactory parameters in this test are usually due to one or more of the following cervical factors: viscous cervical mucus, chronic endocervitis, and cervical stenosis. Vaginal abnormalities affecting the results include narrowing of the introitus, vaginismus, faulty sexual technique, endometriosis, and pelvic inflammatory diseases. Immunologic factors which may affect sperm viability and motility are antibodies in the cervical mucus to the blood group antigens in the sperm. If the above features fail to identify a mechanical, obstructive, or immunologic defect as the cause of infertility, then it is important to determine the integrity of other factors in the female. It is essential to determine whether the following phases of the menstrual cycle are intact: (1) FSH secretion, follicular maturation, estrogen secretion, and endometrial proliferation; (2) LH secretion and ovulation; and (3) corpus luteum function, progesterone production, and secretory endometrial changes. Evaluation of these phases of the cycle was previously considered in Chapter 6 and will, therefore, be presented in summary form here. The recommended clinical observations to establish the existence of these phases of the cycle are: (1) basal body temperature; (2) cyclic vaginal cytologic changes; (3) quality of cervical mucus; (4) endometrial changes on at least 3 specimens taken at 2-wk intervals; and (5) progesterone withdrawal test.

1. Biphasic basal body temperature curves consisting of 0.7–1°F temperature elevations lasting for 13–14 days reflect the presence of progesterone and, therefore, of prior ovulation. Such patterns observed over a course of 3–4 mo would be consistent with normal ovulation.

2. Vaginal cytology reflects estrogen and progesterone effects quite closely, and observations of such cyclic changes would suggest normal ovulation pattern.

3. Persistent ferning of cervical mucus indicates estrogen effect and the absence or deficiency of progesterone.

4. Lack of secretory changes in all of 3 endometrial biopsy specimens taken at 2-wk intervals is consistent with absence of normal cycles and decreased progesterone effect.

5. Absence of withdrawal bleeding after a progesterone challenge suggests deficient estrogen priming, endometrial nonresponsiveness, or pregnancy.

Additional studies are designed to determine the integrity of the hypo-thalamic-pituitary-ovarian axis as outlined under the discussion on amenor-rhea. Procedures for diagnosis of hypergonadotropic hypogonadism include quantitation of plasma FSH and LH (see Chapter 6). Confirmation of diag-nosis of hypogonadotropic hypogonadism as a cause of infertility requires challenges to the anterior pituitary by the FSH/LH-RH, and to the hypothala-mus by clomiphene as detailed previously. Lack of FSH and LH elevations after a challenge with FSH/LH-RH is diagnostic of hypogonadotropinism. Lack of response to clomiphene in the presence of normal response to FSH/LH-RH would implicate a hypothalamic defect. It is essential that other functions of the pituitary should be evaluated before making a diagnosis of isolated hypogonadotropinism. Accordingly, the simultaneous combined chal-lenges with insulin hypoglycemia, TRF, and FSH/LH-RH, as detailed previ-ously, is recommended.

Disorders of the adrenal cortex often cause infertility by disturbance of the feedback regulation of the ovarian-hypothalamic axis. Production of excessive amounts of biosynthetic intermediates in Cushing's syndrome, or of testosterone (and estradiol) in certain biosynthetic defects, interferes with hypothalamic regulation. Evaluation of the adrenal in infertility problems depends on associated clinical stigmata which reflect the types of steroids produced in excess. The definitive methods have been described in detail in another section. Of special interest are quantitation of urinary 17-KGS, 17-KS, 17-OHCS, THS, THDOC, THB, and, pregnanetriol and their responses to appropriate stimulatory and suppression procedures, as well as plasma cortisol, testosterone, pregnanetriol, 11-deoxycortisol, and 11-desoxycortico-sterone levels. The mechanism of disturbed ovulation which occasionally occurs in adrenocortical insufficiency is not clear, but it has been ascribed to the inanition and secondary disturbance in pituitary function. Plasma cortisol levels before and after cosyntropin stimulation is a reliable test for adrenocor-tical insufficiency.

Menstrual cyclicity, ovulation, and infertility may be disturbed by both hyperthyroid and hypothyroid disorders (fig. 7.2). The tests utilized in the diagnosis of these diseases include T_4 levels, free T_4 index, T_3 levels, epithyroid ^{131}I uptake, serum TSH levels, and, occasionally, tanned red cell agglutination studies for thyroglobulin antibodies. These studies are described in greater detail in another section. It is essential that other systemic disorders be considered in the workup of infertility due to disturbed menstrual cycles. For this purpose, complete history and physical examination, as well as the various procedures recommended under the discussion of amenorrhea, may be necessary. It is essential in all cases to diagnose and manage life-threatening illnesses.

HORMONAL METHODS OF CONTRACEPTION

Various social and socioeconomic factors have prompted the use of methods of humane population control in several areas of the world. The hormonal methods of contraception have enjoyed widespread use especially in the western world. Five types of systemic contraceptive agents are in widespread use now. They are: (1) combined estrogen-progestogen pills; (2) sequential estrogen-progestogen pills; (3) the "mini pills" of progestogens; (4) injectable long-acting contraceptives; and (5) the postcoital or "morning after" pills. The mechanisms of actions and success of these regimens differ considerably, but all of these agents alter the hormonal events controlling either the process of ovulation, sperm migration, or tubular transport and implantation of the ovum.

1. The combined estrogen-progestogen pills contain an estrogen combined with a progestational hormone and are given for a fixed number of days, usually 20–24, then discontinued to permit withdrawal bleeding, and reinstated. The several combinations employed and the duration of administration are presented in table 7.3. This method of hormonal therapy inhibits normal secretion of FSH and LH, with resultant failure of ovulation. Extensive statistical studies reveal a pregnancy rate of $< 1:1,000$ women-years with the use of this regimen.

2. The sequential contraceptives are given as estrogens alone for 15–20 days, followed by combined estrogens and progestogens for 5 days. The hormones act on the hypophysiotropic area of the hypothalamus to disturb the secretion of FSH and LH by the anterior pituitary. This sequence is characterized by persistently low levels of plasma FSH and multiple spikes of LH. The persistent suppression of FSH is followed by failure of development of the active principle of the ovary, the follicle. The use of this sequential method of conception control has resulted in a pregnancy rate of about $5:1,000$ women-years.

Both of the above methods may be associated with undesired side-effects, which are ascribed mainly to the estrogen components. There are convincing data that thrombophlebitis and embolic phenomena may occur as a result of use of high estrogen-containing pills. The incidence of these complications presumably decreases with smaller doses of estrogens (Council on Drugs, 1970). Crane, Harris, and Windsor (1971) have provided convincing data on the incidence of hypertension in patients receiving estrogens for contraception. The mechanism of this action probably involves the increased availability of angiotensinogen for angiotensin synthesis. Haggard et al. (1969) reported hyperlipidemia following the use of these agents.

3. The "mini pills" contain microgram amounts of 17-acetoxy derivatives of

Table 7.3. Oral Contraceptive Agents in Common Use

Agent	Manufacturer	Estrogen (mg)	Progestogen (mg)
Combination type[a]			
Enovid-5	Searle	Mestranol (75)	Norethynodrel (5)
Enovid-E	Searle	Mestranol (100)	Norethynodrel (2.5)
Ovulen	Searle	Mestranol (100)	Ethynodiol dracetate (1)
Demulen	Searle	Ethinylestradiol (50)	Ethynodiol dracetate (1)
Norinyl-2	Syntex	Mestranol (100)	Norethindrone (2)
Norinyl 1/50	Syntex	Mestranol (50)	Norethindrone (1)
Norinyl 1/80	Syntex	Mestranol (80)	Norethindrone (1)
Norlestrin 2.5	Parke-Davis	Ethinyl estradiol (50)	Norethindrone acetate (2.5)
Norlestrin 1	Parke-Davis	Ethinyl estradiol (50)	Norethindrone acetate (2.5)
Ortho-Novum 10	Ortho	Mestranol (60)	Norethindrone (10)
Ortho-Novum 2	Ortho	Mestranol (100)	Norethindrone (2)
Ortho-Novum 1/50	Ortho	Mestranol (50)	Norethindrone (1)
Ortho-Novum 1/80	Ortho	Mestranol (80)	Norethindrone (1)
Ovral	Wyeth	Ethinyl estradiol (50)	Norgestrel (0.5)
Sequential type[b]			
Norquen	Syntex	Mestranol (80)	Norethindrone (2)
Ortho-Novum SQ	Ortho	Mestranol (80)	Norethindrone (2)
Oracon	Mead Johnson	Ethinylestradiol (100)	Dimethesterone (25)
Progestogen only			
NOR Q.D.	Syntex		Norethindrone (350)
Micronor	Ortho		Norethindrone (350)

[a]Combination type pills are taken from day 5 through 24 or 25 of the cycle, or 21 days of treatment followed by 7 days of no pill or inert pills.
[b]In sequential type pills, estrogens are taken for first 14–16 days of cycle and for the subsequent 5 or 6 days a combination is taken.

progesterone and some 19-nortestosterone derivatives. These agents presumably inhibit sperm movement through the cervical mucus. The use of this regimen avoids the complications associated with methods (1) and (2) above, but there may be a relatively high occurrence of intermenstrual bleeding and amenorrhea.

4. Of the long-acting hormonal contraceptives, depo-medroxyprogesterone is the most widely employed. The drug is given at a dose level of 150 mg intramuscularly every 3 months. This dosage prevents ovulation and inhibits uterine receptiveness and sperm penetration. Plasma levels of FSH, LH, and estrogens remain in the low ranges of the follicular phase of the menstrual cycle. This regimen is accompanied by a relatively high incidence of irregular bleeding and prolonged amenorrhea after discontinuation of the drug.

5. Postcoital administration of diethylstilbestrol (25 mg twice daily for 5 days begun within 72 hr of intercourse) has been highly successful as a conception preventive. This dosage of synthetic estrogen presumably accelerates tubal transport of the fertilized ovum to an unprepared endometrium with resulting nonimplantation. Many patients complain of nausea, vomiting, and abdominal pain with the use of this dose of diethylstilbestrol.

Amenorrhea Due to Prolonged Use of Oral Contraceptives

There are now considerable data indicating that secondary amenorrhea is frequently found in patients withdrawn from oral contraceptive pills (the postpill amenorrhea syndrome). Approximately 4% of women taking such agents may have this disorder, and the phenomenon is apparently unrelated to duration or type of medication. In one survey of this type of disorder, it was suggested that antecedent history of menstrual disorders is important. Patients with this syndrome have a strong tendency for spontaneous remission. It was suggested that patients with suppression of the cyclic hypothalamic center may require clomiphene stimulation for restitution of cycles and ovulation, whereas those with suppression of the tonic center may require substitution estrogen therapy to avoid atrophy of the genital organs.

REFERENCES

Bacchus, H. 1972. Endocrine profiles in the clinical laboratory. *In* M. Stefanini (ed.), Progress in Clinical Pathology. Vol IV. Grune & Stratton, Inc., New York. pp. 1–101.

Behrman, S. J., and R. W. Kistner (eds.). 1968. Progress in Infertility. Little, Brown & Company, Boston.

Council on Drugs. 1970. Contraceptives J.A.M.A. 214:2316–2321.

Crane, M. J., J. J. Harris, and W. Windsor. 1971. Hypertension, oral contraceptive agents, and conjugated estrogens. Ann. Int. Med. 74:13–21.

Haggard, W. R., M. J. Spiger, J. D. Bagdade, and E. L. Bierman. 1969. Studies on the mechanism of increased plasma triglyceride levels induced by oral contraceptives. New England J. Med. 280:471–475.

Israel, S. L. 1967. Menstrual Disorders and Sterility. Harper & Row, Publishers, New York.

Vande Wiele, R. L. 1972. Treatment of infertility due to ovulatory failure. Hospital Pract. 7:119–131.

8

The
Breasts

The breasts constitute integral parts of the female reproductive system and function under similar endocrine influences as the other secondary sexual organs (Tanner, 1969; Root, 1973*a*; Root, 1973*b*). There are considerable species differences in the responses of these tissue to the gonadal hormones, but most studies indicate that breast development requires the presence of anterior pituitary hormones, and, therefore, of the hypothalamic-pituitary axis. There are data to indicate that pituitary growth hormone, cortisol, and thyroid hormone undoubtedly play permissive roles in the effects of gonadal hormones on breast tissue. It is also probable that some of the effects of these nongonadal hormones relate to their influence of intermediary energy metabolism.

In the presence of the permissive factors listed above, estrogens stimulate the development, elongation, and thickening of the ductal system in the breasts. Progesterone then induces the formation of buds in the distal parts of the ducts. This budding process precedes the eventual formation of breast alveoli. Despite the purported pituitary dependence of the above processes, experimental studies have shown that placental hormones may substitute for the pituitary presence in the pregnant rat.

MATURATION OF DUCTAL AND LOBULE-ALVEOLAR SYSTEM

From birth until the time of puberty, the breast is made up of a group of straight tubules of ectodermal origin which gradually undergo lengthening. A significant spurt of development takes place at the time of puberty correlating with the spurt of pituitary-ovarian activity. The stages of breast development in the female subject have been extensively studied by Marshall and Tanner (1969), and are summarized in table 8.1. (See also fig. 5.1.)

Table 8.1. Stages of Breast Growth in Females

Stage	Features	Age of onset (yr)
1	Prepubertal	
2	Breast budding, widening of are-ola, with elevation upon mound of subareolar tissue; presence of erect papilla	8.9–13.3
3	Enlargement of breast and areolar widening without separation of their contours	10–14.3
4	Projection of areola and papilla above plane of enlarging breast	10.8–15.3
5	Mature breast, erect papilla, are-ola and breast in same plane	11.9–18.8

CYCLIC CHANGES IN THE BREAST

Cyclic changes, essentially synchronous with the menstrual cycle, are observed in the female breast. Animal studies have demonstrated epithelial cyclic changes in the breast, but such observations have not been definitely confirmed in the human female. Nevertheless, the fact that there is cyclic breast engorgement is established. This physiologic engorgement which is ascribed to edema and hyperemia of the lobule-alveolar system is manifested by swelling, tenderness, and, in many women, pain during the premenstruum. This pattern of premenstrual breast engorgement is especially marked for a few years prior to the menopause, and occurs less frequently if the patient has had several pregnancies.

Cyclic breast changes are often difficult to differentiate from cystic disease since as many as 20% of women between age 25 and the menopause have gross cystic disease (defined as palpable masses). Occasionally, differentiation from carcinomatous processes is difficult. In general, physiologic engorgement is associated with diffuse nodularity most evident in the upper quadrants of the breasts. Carcinoma is characterized usually by a dominant single tumor without a predilection for the upper halves of the breasts.

BREAST CHANGES DURING PREGNANCY

Enlargement of the breasts with considerable increase of the lobule-alveolar structures occur during pregnancy. These changes are ascribed to the increased amounts of estrogens and progesterone, as well as other hormones from the placenta. After full breast development, the production of milk is induced by the pituitary hormone prolactin (PRL). Elevated levels of PRL appear during pregnancy by the eighth week of gestation and continue to rise to values of 200 ng/ml at term. In the absence of breast feeding, the levels return to normal (around 10 ng/ml) within 2–3 wk. There are characteristic responses in serum prolactin in women who breast feed their babies. Early in the postpartum period, 30-min suckling is followed by a modest increase in PRL. From the second to the twelfth weeks postpartum, basal PRL levels are around 20 ng/ml, but the same suckling stimulus is now followed by a 10- to 20-fold increase of PRL. After 12–16 wk, the basal PRL levels are again normal and fail to respond to the suckling stimulus (Tyson, Hwang, and Guyda, 1972). Initiation of lactation by prolactin is dependent on the levels of estrogens and progesterone. According to the double threshold theory of Folley, low levels of estrogens activate the lactogenic function of the pituitary, but higher levels inhibit the process. While certain critical low estrogen levels activate release of prolactin by suppressing the release of PIF from the hypothalamus, suitable amounts of progesterone inhibit this activation. It is probable that the high progesterone levels in pregnancy inhibit lactation. The decreased levels of progesterone occurring at the time of delivery remove this inhibition and, as a result, the release of prolactin by estrogen alone occurs. While PRL is essential for lactation, the presence of GH and adrenal steroids enhance the process.

HPL achieves measurable levels at about 6 wk gestation and reaches peak levels of 6,000 ng/ml at term (Fournier, Desjardins, and Friesen, 1974). Despite the fact that both PRL and HPL serve lactogenic functions, this activity occurs only after parturition. The lactogenic functions of both hormones are undoubtedly inhibited by ovarian and placental steroids. Experimental studies have confirmed the concept that the activation of lactation in the postpartum period is suppressed by exogenous estrogens, probably because they block the peripheral action of HPL.

Stimulation of PRL release by TRH is followed by breast engorgement within 2–3 hr. Analysis of milk obtained from these stimulated breasts revealed significant increased levels of protein and fat. These data suggest that prolactin stimulates the synthesis of protein and lipids by the mammary glands (Fournier, Desjardins, and Friesen, 1974).

Surges of PRL which follow the suckling stimulus are responsible for alterations in the secretion and release of the gonadotropins FSH and LH. Women who breast feed their babies have more prolonged amenorrhea, nonovulatory cycles, and infertility than women who do not. Some studies suggest that this is due to a lack of responsiveness of the ovaries to FSH and LH in women who breast feed. In addition there are data which reveal that the FSH and LH responses to FSH/LH-RH challenges are subnormal in

Table 8.2. Factors Affecting Serum Prolactin Levels

I. Causes of increased prolactin
  A. Physiologic and drugs
    1. Suckling, stress, hypoglycemia
    2. Increased osmolality
    3. TRH
    4. Estrogens
    5. α-methyldopa
    6. Phenothiazines
    7. Reserpine, tricyclic antidepressants
  B. Pathologic states
    1. Prolactin-secreting tumors of pituitary (25% of all pituitary tumors)
      a) With galactorrhea
      b) Without galactorrhea
    2. Hypothalamic lesions with resulting decreased PIF
      a) Functional (Chiari Frommel)
      b) Organic (tumor)
    3. Pituitary stalk section
    4. Hypothyroidism
    5. Ectopic production
    6. Renal failure (10–20% of patients)

II. Causes of decreased prolactin levels
  A. Decreased serum osmolality
  B. Hyperglycemia
  C. L-dopa
  D. Ergocryptine

patients who lactate. It is, therefore, likely that the periodic elevations of PRL which follow suckling exert an inhibitory effect both on the pituitary and on the response of the ovaries.

Several lines of data indicate that prolactin stimulates metabolic activity in the mammary glands by formation of cyclic adenosine monophosphate from ATP. It has also been demonstrated that PRL interacts with receptors in the cell membrane of the mammary cell, but the activation of membrane adenyl cyclase has not yet been proved.

Several physiologic, pathologic, and chemical factors influence the release of PRL by the anterior pituitary (table 8.2), and many of these may underlie some of the clinical entities characterized by inappropriate lactation. It is also clear now that, despite the role of PRL in initiating lactation, elevated PRL is not invariably associated with lactation. Similarly inappropriate lactation has occurred in patients without demonstrable PRL elevations.

SYNDROMES OF INAPPROPRIATE LACTATION (GALACTORRHEA)

Inappropriate lactation or pathologic galactorrhea refers to the presence of secretion of breast milk inappropriate to the physiologic state of the individual. Differentiation from appropriate lactation (as occurs immediately postpartum) is important since several pathologic and physiologic aberrations may underlie its occurrence. The lactation seen in the newborn is ascribed to a temporary secretion of prolactin by the baby's own pituitary, but the plethora of maternal prolactin and placental HPL have been implicated in its development. Table 8.3 presents the various causes of inappropriate lactation along with data on the presence of hyperprolactinemia and the probable mechanism of development. It is noted that several types of galactorrhea are characterized by hyperprolactinemia, whereas in others there is no such correlation. This observation is consistent with considerations presented above on the factors which affect prolactin secretion. It is clear that factors which suppress the release of hypothalamic neurohormone PIF permit the release of PRL by the pituitary. Similarly, factors which influence TRH release by the hypothalamus induce release of PRL. In addition to the chemical influences on hypothalamic neurohormone release, several mechanical factors, such as disturbance of the portal system to the pituitary, and pathologic processes, such as tumors and postinfectious states, may affect transport of the neurohormones to the pituitary. In still other disorders, the pathogenesis of the galactorrhea is not clear. Amenorrhea occurs quite frequently in the lactation syndrome, and is often ascribed to a shift in pituitary hormone production to excess prolactin secretion. This explanation is undoubtedly inadequate for the amenorrhea which occurs in the absence of elevated prolactin.

An eponymic classification of inappropriate lactation syndromes into the Chiari-Frommel (postpartum), the Ahumada-Argonz-del Castillo, and Forbes-Albright syndromes has been presented in several articles. This classification is of questionable value and, indeed, may be quite misleading in understanding the pathogenesis of these disorders. Indeed, cases have been described which have evolved through all three syndromes (Mahesh, Dalla Pria, and Greenblatt, 1969), while others have eventually developed Cushing's disease or acromegaly. The classification is presented in table 8.4 largely because of its presence in standard texts (American College of Physicians, 1974) and not because of its intrinsic usefulness.

Diagnostic Investigation of Galactorrhea

Definitive investigation of inappropriate lactation syndromes presumes cognizance of the several etiologic factors. It is, therefore, essential that a

Table 8.3. Causes of Inappropriate Lactation

Disorder	Hyperprolactinemia	Mechanism
Pathologic states		
Pituitary tumors		
Cushing's disease	?	
Acromegaly	+	Unknown; GH may be involved
"Nonfunctioning" adenoma	+	Autonomous PRL secretion
Hypopituitarism		
Idiopathic		
Post-traumatic		
Postpartum necrosis (Sheehan's)		
After pituitary stalk section	+	Absence of tonc inhibition by PIF
Post-encephalitis		
Encephalitis basal meningitis		
Pinealoma		
Primary hypothyroidism		
With amenorrhea	+	TRH release of PRL
With sexual precocity		
Hyperthyroidism		
Estrogen-secreting tumor		
Nonendocrine tumors	+	Ectopic PRL secretion
Local Factors		
Thoracic surgery		
Thoracic cage surgery		
Herpes zoster of chest wall		
Pharmacologic agents		
Phenothiazines	+	Inhibition of hypothalamic release of PIF by the agents listed
Oral contraceptive agents	+	
Estrogens	+	
Reserpine	+	
α-Methyldopa	+	
Perphenazine	+	
Imipramine	+	

Table 8.4. Eponymic Classification of Inappropriate Lactation

	Chiari-Frommel	del Castillo	Forbes-Albright
Onset[a]	Postpartum	Spontaneous	Postpartum or spontaneous
Sella turcica	Normal	Normal	Enlarged
Natural history[b]	Usually transitory	Usually permanent	Permanent

[a]The del Castillo type is often ascribable to pharmacologic agents.
[b]Progression from one type to another has been described (see text).

complete history, with special emphasis on menses, pregnancy, and details of drug ingestion, be obtained. A complete physical examination is essential to determine the presence of stigmata diagnostic of several of the etiologic causes, *e.g.*, chest injury, acromegaly, and Cushing's syndrome among others. Laboratory studies should include the following tests. (1) X-ray studies of the skull, in appropriate views for sella turcica volume determination. An air encephalogram should be done if indicated by visual field defects, or by diabetes insipidus. (2) Anterior pituitary function studies are necessary to determine integrity of the axes to the adrenals, thyroid, and gonads, as well as GH release. The definitive studies have been described in Chapters 3 and 6. These may be conveniently assessed by the combined pituitary challenge described elsewhere. Hypothalamic release of LH/FSH-RH is assessed by the clomiphene challenge test. (3) Thyroid functions are assessed by measurement of T_4 resin uptake of T_3, T_3 by radioimmunoassay (if hyperthyroidism is a diagnostic possibility), TSH levels before and after TRH (if needed), and thyroglobulin antibodies. These procedures are detailed in Chapter 9.

Differentiation of the hyperprolactinemia associated with pituitary tumors from that due to benign disorders by the L-dopa challenge has not proved very reliable (Turkington, 1972). The water loading test (Buckman et al., 1973) was quite effective in differentiating the two types of hyperprolactinemia. The procedure employs the principle that induction of hypoosmolarity is followed by a > 50% decrease of prolactin in normal individuals and in patients with functional hyperprolactinemia. Significant decreases are not found in patients with hyperprolactinemia due to pituitary tumors.

Natural History of Galactorrhea Syndromes

The natural history of these disorders depends on the nature of the underlying causes. Several types may be of a transient nature and disappear spontaneously. Others evolve into manifestations of the underlying disorders. Pituitary tumors may progress quite insidiously before there is clinical or laboratory evidence of an intracranial neoplasm. Visual defects, pituitary apoplexy, cardiomyopathy, and abnormal carbohydrate and lipid metabolism are among the more serious consequences of untreated acromegaly, although in many patients the process may become "burnt out." The prognosis in Cushing's syndrome is basically quite poor unless treated; congestive heart failure, hypertensive disease, severe osteoporosis with vertebrae collapse and cord interruption are among the more ominous sequelae. The natural history of untreated hyperthyroidism is described in another section. Inappropriate lactation due to drug ingestion is usually reversible on cessation of the agents, but the galactorrhea due to oral contraceptive agents may persist after their discontinuation. As pointed out above, patients with galactorrhea ascribed to the Chiari Frommel syndrome have later been found to have pituitary tumors or other intracranial neoplasms.

Treatment of Galactorrhea Syndromes

Emphasis in the management of these disorders is directed to the underlying causes, of which inappropriate lactation is a reflection. Patients with drug-induced galactorrhea improve merely by discontinuation of the drugs responsible. However, the inappropriate lactation occasionally associated with ingestion of oral contraceptive agents may persist quite beyond their discontinuation. Many of these patients may ovulate and show subsequent disappearance of the galactorrhea after being treated with clomiphene for ovulation. The galactorrhea which is seen in patients on phenothiazines and similar drugs usually disappears on cessation of the inciting agents. The use of L-dopa to restimulate PIF production is occasionally helpful, but the response is not sustained.

Galactorrhea which follows local chest trauma regresses spontaneously. Appropriate treatment of thyroid disorders (see Chapter 10) is usually followed by permanent remission of the galactorrhea. Disorders of the hypothalamus and pituitary which are manifested by galactorrhea are difficult to treat. Definitive surgery for pituitary tumors is recommended when there are visual field defects, but this method may exacerbate the galactorrhea since remaining pituitary cells may be completely separated from the inhibitory influence of PIF from the hypothalamus. Pituitary irradiation is rarely followed by improvement of amenorrhea and galactorrhea. Patients without any evidence of intracranial tumors have been tried on treatment with estrogens and progesterone, but without good results. The ergot alkaloid 2-Br-α-ergocryptine relieves the galactorrhea, often within a few days, and apparently has a sustained effect. Patients treated with this medication have a return of menses, and the pituitary responsiveness to clomiphene returns to normal. This drug is also useful in management of the galactorrhea observed after the use of oral contraceptive agents, and in the Chiari-Frommel syndrome. The drug suppresses the release of prolactin by the pituitary and this suppression of prolactin presumably permits gonadotropin release.

HORMONAL EFFECTS ON BREAST CANCER

Development of the normal breast has been shown to depend on an intricate interplay between estrogens and progesterone in the permissive milieu accomodated by thyroid hormone, growth hormone, and cortisol. The participation of prolactin in milk production has been discussed. There are now several lines of data which indicate that an interplay between estrogen progesterone and prolactin is intimately involved with neoplastic growth in the breast. Prolactin has been shown in experimental studies to significantly influence the growth of breast tumors. Prolactin, even in the absence of the ovaries, adrenals, and pituitary, has been shown to reactivate mammary tumors in experimental animals (Pearson et al., 1969). Tumor regression was noted after the use of antiprolactin serum in experimental animals (Butler and Pearson, 1971). Pharmacologic agents, such as ergocornine, which inhibit prolactin secretion have inhibited experimental breast tumor growths (Quadri and Meites, 1971). Clinical studies on human breast cancer have suggested a central role of the pituitary in the progression of tumor growth (McGuire et al., 1974). This effect is presumably mediated by prolactin. Recent studies have demonstrated that the bone pain secondary to bony metastasis from breast cancer is relieved with the use of L-dopa (Minton, 1974). This agent suppresses the release of prolactin inhibitory factor. On the other hand, there are some studies suggesting that pituitary stalk section, which should increase prolactin release, is followed by human breast tumor regression.

Estrogens stimulate normal breast growth and differentiation. Data indicating that estrogens fail to support breast tumor growth in the absence of the pituitary have been interpreted as evidence that the role of estrogens in breast tumorigenesis is a secondary one. The mechanism of estrogen action on target cells has been discussed in Chapter 1. It has been suggested by several experimental studies that, in breast tissue, the estrogen-cytosol receptor reactions and subsequent steps may also affect the actions of other steroid (e.g., progesterone and testosterone) receptors in the cytosol, as well as possibly the cell membrane receptivity to prolactin. Experimental studies suggest the absence of estrogen receptor in autonomous breast tumors. This loss has been interpreted as evidence of at least a partial disintegration of the endocrine regulatory unit of the breast tissue. It has been suggested that the presence of estrogen receptor in breast tumors would suggest hormone dependence and, therefore, be of predictive value in the responsiveness to hormonal manipulation (McGuire et al., 1974).

REFERENCES

American College of Physicians. 1974. Medical knowledge self-assessment program. III. Recent developments in internal medicine. p. 28.

144   Habeeb Bacchus

Buckman, M. T., N. Kaminsky, M. Conway, and G. T. Peake. 1973. Utility of
L-dopa and water loading in evaluation of hyperprolactinemia. J. Clin.
Endocrinol. 36:911—919.

Butler, T. P., and O. H. Pearson. 1971. Regression of prolactin-dependent rat
mammary carcinoma in response to anti-hormone treatment. Cancer Res.
31:817.

Fournier, P. J. R., P. D. Desjardins, and H. G. Friesen. 1974. Current
understanding of human prolactin physiology and its diagnostic and therapeutic implications. Am. J. Obst. & Gynec. 118:337—343.

Mahesh, V. B., S. Dalla Pria, and R. B. Greenblatt. 1969. Abnormal lactation
with Cushing's syndrome. J. Clin. Endocrinol. 29:978—981.

Marshall, W. A., and J. M. Tanner. 1969. Variations in pattern of pubertal
changes in girls. Arch. Dis. Childhood 44:291—303.

McGuire, W. L., G. C. Chamners, M. E. Costlow, and R. E. Shepherd. 1974.
Hormone dependence in breast cancer. Metabolism 23:75—99.

Minton, J. P. 1974. The response of breast cancer patients with bone pains to
L-dopa. Cancer 33:358—363.

Pearson, O. H., O. Llerena, L. Llerena, and. 1969. Prolactin-dependent
mammary cancer: A model for man? Tr. A. Am. Physicians 82:255.

Quadri, S. K., and J. Meites. 1971. Regression of spontaneous mammary
tumors in rats by ergot drugs. Proc. Soc. Exper. Biol. & Med. 138:999—1001.

Root, A. W. 1973. Endocrinology of puberty. I. Normal sexual maturation. J.
Pediat. 83:1—19.

Root, A. W. 1973. Endocrinology of puberty. II. Aberrations of sexual
maturation. J. Pediat. 83:187—200.

Tanner, J. M. 1969. Growth and endocrinology of the adolescent. In L. I.
Gardner (ed.), Endocrine and Genetic Diseases of Childhood, pp. 19—76. W.
B. Saunders Company, Philadelphia.

Turkington, R. W. 1972. Inhibition of prolactin secretion and successful
therapy of the Forbes-Albright syndrome with L-dopa. J. Clin. Endocrinol.
34:306—311.

Tyson, J. E., P. Hwang, H. Guyda. 1972. Studies of prolactin secretion in
human pregnancy. Am. J. Obst. & Gynec. 113:14—20.

9

The
Thyroid
Gland

Several aspects of the female reproductive cycle are influenced by the thyroid gland through its hormones thyroxin (T_4) and triiodothyronine (T_3) (Ingbar and Woeber, 1969; Werner and Ingbar, 1971; Rawson, Money, and Grief, 1969; Tata, 1964). The thyroid gland consists of two lobes joined by an isthmus and attached to the anterior aspect of the trachea. The weight of the gland in the adult is 15–20 g. The embryologic origin of the medial part of the gland is from the pharyngeal floor at the level of the first and second pouches; the lateral areas are derived from the fourth pouches. Evidence of thyrogenesis is first seen at the seventeenth gestation day. It is assumed that in the evolutionary scale this gland served an exocrine function. At maturity, this gland stores its hormonal products in colloid-containing vesicles enclosed by epithelium, and, in this respect, this endocrine gland is unique. The thyroglobulin in the vesicles contains the iodinated compounds, iodotyrosines, which are monoiodotyrosine (MIT), diiodotyrosine (DIT), and the iodothyronines, namely, triiodothyronine (T_3) and thyroxin (tetraiodothyronine, T_4). In close anatomic relationship to the thyroid are the four parathyroids which are derived from the third and fourth branchial arches. The hormone produced by the parathyroids, parathyroid hormone (PTH), is involved in calcium and bone metabolism. Parafollicular cells or C cells associated with the thyroid gland are derived from the sixth branchial arch. These cells produce the hormone calcitonin which retards bone resorption.

Early development of the thyroid gland is independent of pituitary but, by the time the gland forms colloid at the thirteenth week, further thyroid development and regulation come under pituitary control through TSH. There is a direct correlation between the height of thyroid follicular cells and the levels of TSH, so that removal of the pituitary support is associated with atrophic changes in the thyroid.

The hormones of the thyroid gland, T_4 and T_3, are synthesized from the substrates tyrosine and iodine. The amino acid tyrosine is present in the thyroglobulin molecule stored in the follicles as colloid, each thyroglobulin molecule containing 115 tyrosyl residues. Strategically located tyrosyls are iodinated in the presence of I^o, whose eventual source is food and water. I^o is reduced to iodide in the gastrointestinal tract where it is rapidly absorbed. Iodide in the blood stream is taken up by the salivary glands, the stomach mucosa, and mammary tissue, but the iodide-trapping mechanism in the thyroid is several times more efficient than the others. Therefore, 90% of total body iodine is concentrated in the thyroid. The thyroid iodine pool, which is mainly organic iodide in thyroglobulin, is 5,000–7,000 μg, and this pool has a turnover rate of 1% daily.

BIOSYNTHESIS OF THYROID HORMONES

The processes involved in hormone synthesis in the thyroid include the following: trapping of iodide; organification of iodine; coupling of iodotyrosines; release of T_3 and T_4 from thyroglobulin; and deiodination of iodotyrosines (fig. 9.1).

Trapping of Iodide

Thyroid iodide trapping is the process of uptake of iodide by the cells of the gland by the iodide pump or iodide trap mechanism. This trapping mechanism has been proved to antedate thyroid follicle development. The process involves concentration of the iodide against strong electric and concentration gradients, with subsequent rapid diffusion of the iodide into the follicular lumen. This process is inhibited by agents such as thiocyanates, perchlorates, nitrites, dinitrophenol, and cardiac glycosides. The requirements for the trapping process are energy, integrity of the cell membranes and of cellular organelles, and the ability to transport Na^+ and K^+ by a system involving Na^+-K^+-dependent ATP-ase. This trapping mechanism is increased by TSH and by iodide ingestion. Iodide is converted to iodine by a thyroid peroxidase system, but possibly other oxidizing systems may also be involved.

Organification of Iodine

In the follicular lumen, spontaneous iodination of certain strategically located accessible tyrosyl moieties in thyroglobulin takes place at or near the surface of the follicle cells. Involvement of an enzymatic (iodinase) system in this process is also possible. This step results in the formation of approximately equal amounts of MIT and DIT under normal conditions. Iodide deficiency is

BIOSYNTHESIS of THYROID HORMONES

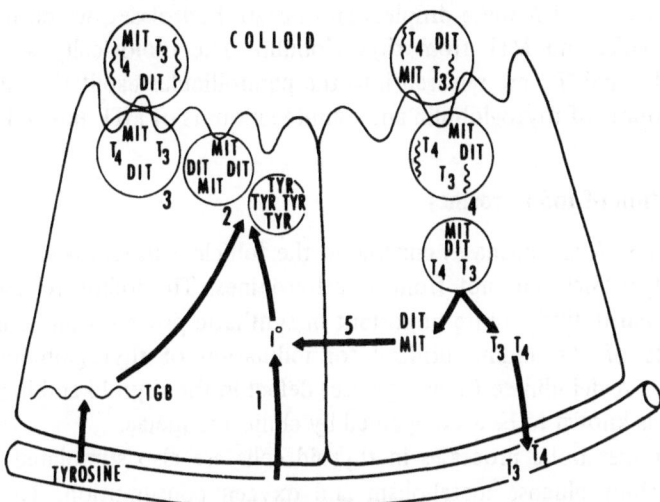

Figure 9.1. Hormone synthesis in the thyroid gland. Steps in the synthesis of thyroxin (T_4) and triiodothyronine (T_3) are depicted. Enzymatic steps are as follows: (1) peroxidase; (2) iodination of tyrosyl moieties (organification of I^O may be nonenzymatic or may be medicated by an iodinase system; (3) the coupling reaction which is probably enzymatic; iodothyronines are synthesized as constituents of thyroglobulin produced on ribosomes and transferred to soluble droplets which are carried to the cell-colloid interface where steps 1 and 2 take place; (4) proteolysis whereby T_4, T_3, diiodotyrosine (DIT), and monoiodotyrosine (MIT) are released from thyroglobulin; and (5) deiodination.

accompanied by a relative decrease in the amount of DIT, with eventual preferential synthesis of T_3, the biologically more powerful hormone. Hence, euthyroidism may be maintained in the face of iodide deficiency. Organification of iodine is blocked by thionamide drugs, such as propylthiouracil and methimazole, agents which are employed in the medical arrangement of hyperthyroidism.

Coupling of Iodotyrosines

MIT and DIT molecules suitably located along thyroglobulin at the cell-colloid interface undergo enzymatic coupling reactions as follows: MIT and DIT to form T_3, and DIT and DIT to form T_4. In iodide deficiency states, the first reaction is predominant, resulting in a relative increase in formation of T_3, which is biologically more active than T_4.

Release of T_3 and T_4 from Thyroglobulin

Release of T_3 and T_4 from thyroglobulin colloid is taken up by epithelial follicular cells by the process of pinocytosis. This step is stimulated by TSH by activation of membrane adenyl cyclase with the release of cAMP. Lysosomes coalesce with these droplets and release hydrolases, which release T_4 and T_3, DIT, and MIT from thyroglobulin. The biologically active compounds T_4 and T_3 are released into the parafollicular capillaries along with small amounts of thyroglobulin and minute amounts of MIT and DIT.

Deiodination of Iodotyrosines

A deiodinase (dehalogenase) enzyme in the follicle cells removes iodine from the iodotyrosines, but not from iodothyronines. The iodine release in this step is quantitatively quite important in synthetic processes and constitutes two-thirds of the iodine utilized for iodination of thyroglobulin tyrosyl molecules. A deiodinase (dehalogenase) defect in the thyroid and in peripheral tissues is known to be accompanied by clinical sequelae.

Other metabolic processes in thyroid cells are also stimulated by TSH. These include glucose metabolism and oxygen consumption. The derived energy and cofactors are essential for thyroid hormonogenesis. TSH action on these parameters is mediated by membrane adenyl cyclase release, which is noted within minutes after TSH administration.

TRANSPORT OF THYROID HORMONES

Both thyroid hormones thyroxin (T_4) and triiodothyronine (T_3) are transported reversibly, but firmly bound, to serum proteins. The major transport substance is thyroid-binding globulin (TBG), which is a glycoprotein with mobility on electrophoresis between α_1 and α_2 regions. Thyroid-binding prealbumin (TBPA) (presumably identical with prealbumin 1) is the second, and albumin the third, protein carrier of thyroid hormones. TBG- and TBPA-binding sites are saturable, whereas those of albumin are not. TBG levels in the serum do not exceed 1 mg/100 ml, possessing the ability to bind 20 μg of T_4/100 ml of serum. TBPA amounts to 30 mg/100 ml of serum, and one mole of T_4 is bound per mole of TBPA. Structural relationships determine the binding affinities of T_4 and T_3 to the binding proteins, and T_3 is not appreciably bound to TBPA. The affinity of T_3 for TBG is weaker than that of T_4 and is, therefore, readily displaced by the latter. Biologic activities, as well as degradation of the thyroid hormones, are influenced by the binding affinities to carriers.

Of circulating T_4, 0.04% exists in the free form and 99.96% is distributed as follows: 60% bound to TBG, 30% to TBPA, and the remainder to albumin. The proportion of free T_3 is 10 times greater than T_4, *i.e.*, 0.4% is free and 99.6% is protein-bound. The rapid onset of action of T_3 probably is due to its looser affinity for protein binding. The intrinsically greater biologic activity of T_3, compared with T_4, is probably not ascribable to differences in binding affinity, however. Plasma levels of free T_4 amount to 3 ng/100 ml, and of free T_3 to about 1.0–1.5 ng/100 ml, normally. Both T_4 and T_3 are biologically active hormones, but there is known to be a significant conversion of T_4 to T_3 by deiodination, accounting for 50% of T_3 in the circulation. In the absence of contaminants, the levels of protein-bound iodine (PBI) represent a measure of T_4 (total), but these values are influenced by alterations in the binding proteins. For example, higher TBG levels are found in pregnancy and after estrogen therapy, with a resulting high PBI; and low TBG and PBI are found in TBG deficiency.

METABOLISM OF THYROID HORMONES

Degradation of T_4 and T_3 is significantly influenced by the binding proteins. By limiting the levels of free T_4 in the circulation, TBG is responsible for a decreased degradation of the hormone. The exchangeable cellular T_4 flux also influences thyroid hormone metabolism. It is estimated that 10% of the T_4 secreted daily is excreted in the bile mainly as free T_4, with a small portion as glucuronide conjugate. The remainder of thyroid hormone degradation takes place in various tissues, especially liver, kidneys, and muscle. The cellular degradation mechanisms include deiodination, which takes place in the target organs, and deamination, transamination, and decarboxylation reactions, which occur after deiodination. In the liver, these cellular degradative reactions take place in the endoplasmic reticulum.

REGULATION OF THYROID ACTIVITY

Two major regulatory mechanisms for thyroid activity are known (Shenkman, 1972). These are the hypothalamic-pituitary-thyroid axis and intrathyroidal autoregulation.

Hypothalamic-Pituitary-Thyroid Axis

Activity of the thyroid gland is controlled by pituitary TSH. This tropic hormone influences thyroid structure and function, including the size and vascularity, the height of the epithelial cells, and the amounts of stored colloid. TSH also stimulates several intrathyroidal metabolic processes, including glucose oxidation, phospholipid synthesis, and RNA synthesis. Release of TSH from the pituitary is in turn dependent on the levels of free T_4 and T_3. The pituitary-thyroid axis is unique in that there is greater intrinsic pituitary control in this system than in the other pituitary-target gland mechanisms. TSH secretion is inversely proportional to the metabolic effects of T_4 and T_3 in the pituitary. The hypothalamus exerts a modulating influence on pituitary TSH secretion through the neurohormone thyrotropin releasing hormone (TRH), but it is not the final regulator of feedback control of the pituitary-thyroid axis.

Intrathyroidal autoregulation

Intrathyroidal mechanisms designed to maintain a relative constancy of hormonal stores within the gland operate essentially independently of TSH. Large amounts of iodide acutely depress the organic binding and coupling reactions within the gland. This response, the Wolff-Chaikoff effect, prevents massive increases in hormone synthesis. An acute extracellular depletion of iodide induces an increase in iodide clearance and uptake by the thyroid. Under chronic conditions, the glandular content of organic iodine is inversely related to the activity of the iodide transport system. The iodide transport mechanism of the thyroid is more responsive to TSH in a gland depleted of iodide than in the gland rich in iodide. Decreased levels of thyroid hormone stores (reflecting decreased synthesis) initiate changes in intrinsic function and in the responses to TSH. These changes are designed to increase thyroid hormone synthesis. When there are increased hormone stores (reflecting increased hormone synthesis) TSH release by the pituitary is inhibited, and the biosynthetic steps are suppressed (fig. 9.2).

METABOLIC EFFECTS OF THYROID HORMONES

Thyroid hormones (T_4 and T_3) affect several metabolic parameters. The presence of the alanyl side chain confers significant biologic activity to the molecule. Replacement of iodine by other halogens is associated with biologic activity, but at a decreased level. The iodines on the T_4 and T_3 structures provide molecular stability and prevent free rotation around the ether oxygen of these iodothyronines, hence, maintaining the configuration necessary for attachment to the target receptors.

A single regulatory reaction has not been found to explain the multiple effects of thyroid hormones, but there are some data which suggest that the primary action is to increase synthesis of mitochondrial RNA with resulting increase in the incorporation of amino acids into mitochondrial proteins. The known metabolic effects of thyroid hormones are:

1. Increase of oxygen consumption and calorigenesis in heart, liver, kidney, and skeletal muscle

2. Increase of activities of several mitochondrial enzymes, including L-α-

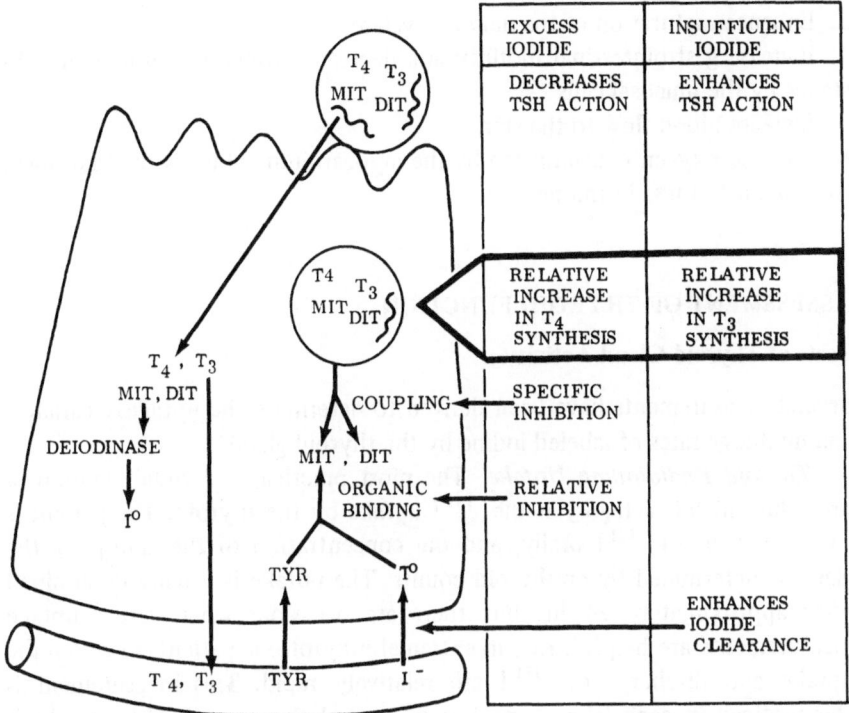

	EXCESS IODIDE	INSUFFICIENT IODIDE
	DECREASES TSH ACTION	ENHANCES TSH ACTION
	RELATIVE INCREASE IN T_4 SYNTHESIS	RELATIVE INCREASE IN T_3 SYNTHESIS
COUPLING	SPECIFIC INHIBITION	
ORGANIC BINDING	RELATIVE INHIBITION	
		ENHANCES IODIDE CLEARANCE

Figure 9.2. Intrathyroidal autoregulation of thyroid hormone synthesis by iodine.

glycerophosphate dehydrogenase which is important in lipid and carbohydrate metabolism

3. Increase of incorporation of amino acids in ribosomes

4. Increase of carbohydrate absorption from the gastrointestinal tract, but decrease of glycogen synthesis

5. Increase of hepatic cholesterologenesis

6. Increase of the excretion of cholesterol into biliary tract

7. Increase of lipolysis and support actions of catecholamines on this activity

8. Increase of renal plasma flow and glomerular filtration rate

9. Increase of bone turnover

10. Required for conversion of carotene to Vitamin A.

The physiologic effects of thyroid hormones are:

1. Increase basal metabolism and oxygen consumption (T_3 is three to four times more powerful than T_4 in increasing oxygen consumption; T_3 is also faster acting in this function)

2. Stimulate and support growth processes in various organs and tissues, e.g., mammary glands and reproductive system

3. Enhance maturation of the nervous system
4. Increase gastrointestinal motility and decrease production of mucoid substance by the mucosal cells
5. Increase blood flow to the skin
6. Increase oxygen consumption by the myocardium, which is the first organ to respond to these hormones

ASSESSMENT OF THYROID FUNCTION

Tests of Thyroid Gland Activity

Several measurements have been derived to determine the uptake, clearance, and discharge rates of labeled iodine by the thyroid gland.

Thyroid Radioiodine Uptake The most practical and widely employed procedure in this category is the ^{131}I uptake by the thyroid. The patient is given 2–15 μc of ^{131}I orally, and the concentration of the isotope in the gland is determined by epithyroid counts. The uptake is usually determined after approximately 24 hr, but there are occasions when earlier uptake measurements are helpful, *e.g.,* in extremely thyrotoxic patients in whom the uptake and discharge of ^{131}I are relatively rapid. This measurement is standardized in each laboratory, but in general the normal 24-hr uptake is between 15–35%. Values below 10% are considered abnormally low and would suggest hypothyroidism. Other disorders characterized by decreased ^{131}I uptake include chronic thyroiditis, subacute (de Quervain's) thyroiditis, iodide trapping defects in the thyroid, acute therapy with antithyroid drugs, and pituitary hypofunction. Other causes, not necessarily associated with thyroid hypofunction, include exogenous iodide (by dilutional effects on iodide pool and by effects on the intrathyroidal regulatory mechanisms), renal and cardiac failure, and, rarely, extreme hyperthyroidism with rapid (before 24 hr) discharge of the labeled iodine.

Epithyroid ^{131}I uptake values greater than 35% are consistent with hyperthyroidism. Other states which may be associated with elevated ^{131}I uptakes include rebound from thyroid suppression, recovery from subacute thyroiditis, and recent withdrawal from an antithyroid drug. In the presence of excess loss of T_4 and T_3, such as in nephrosis, chronic diarrhea, and spontaneous or induced malabsorption states, the thyroid ^{131}I uptake may be high. It is also possible that in a biosynthetic defect, such as in some forms of Hashimoto's thyroiditis, that the ^{131}I uptake may be high because of synthesis and discharge of abnormal iodoproteins.

Triiodothyronine Suppression of Increased Thyroid Radioiodide Uptake Euthyroid individuals given 50–75 μg of T_3 daily for 5–7 days exhibit a significant suppression of their normal thyroid radioiodide uptake. Patients with diffuse toxic goiter fail to show a suppression of their elevated radioiodide uptake after similar T_3 therapy. This test has been especially useful in the diagnosis of T_3 toxicosis patients in whom the baseline radioiodine uptake is often normal.

The Perchlorate or Thiocyanate Washout Test This test is useful in detecting defects in biosynthetic pathways, induced or congenital, in the thyroid. If the iodide-trapping mechanism is intact, then the thyroid radio-iodide uptake appears normal. Radioactivity in the gland is measured after either perchlorate or thiocynate is given orally; uptake readings are made at 60 and 100 min. A decrease of 10% or more of the uptake at 60 min is considered as diagnostic of an error in organic binding of iodine and may be noted in patients with congenital hypothyroidism due to peroxidase defect, in iodide goiter, in thionamide-induced organification defect, in Hashimoto's thyroiditis, in radioiodine treated thyrotoxicosis, and, occasionally, in severe thyrotoxicosis.

The TSH Stimulation Test The TSH stimulation test is most useful in eva-luating findings of a law RAI uptake. After the baseline RAI uptake study, the patient is given 5–10 units of TSH intramuscularly for 3 days (or 1 day occa-sionally). If on repeat RAI uptake, there is no increase, then primary hypo-thyroidism is likely. Normal individuals exhibit an increment in RAI uptake of at least 15% above the baseline. Patients with pituitary hypothyroidism will often show an even greater increment. (Serum T_4 or PBI determinations may also be performed before and after TSH stimulation.)

Thyroid Uptake of Pertechnate ^{99m}TC The pertechnate ion is trapped by the thyroid, but it does not undergo organic binding. The nucleide is given intravenously and epithyroid counts are made up to 30 min after administra-tion. Maximal epithyroid counts are noted in about 20 min. Normal indi-viduals show values less than 2% at this interval. Thyrotoxic patients exhibit an uptake of 5–25% in 20 min. Values in this range may also be found in iodine deficiency and biosynthetic defects in the thyroid (dyshormonogenesis and autoimmune thyroiditis).

Tests of Thyroid Hormones in Blood

Quantitation of iodine attached to proteins has been employed to assay thyroid function on the assumption that most circulating thyroxin is protein-bound. Other newer methods include the quantitation of T_4 and T_3 by radioimmunoassay.

Protein-Bound Iodine Protein-bound iodine determination involves pre-cipitating the serum proteins, digestion or ashing of the precipitate, and determination of the iodine in the precipitate. Normal values of PBI range from 4–8 μ/100 ml. Patients with hyperthyroidism usually have PBI values of greater than 10 μg/100 ml. Newborn babies show PBI values up to 12 μg/100 ml between 5–7 days of life and between 4–8 μg/100 ml later. The method does not eliminate inorganic or organic iodides ingested in medications, foods, or employed in tests. For this reason, values of PBI greater than 25 μg/100 ml should be viewed with suspicion for the probability of contamination. Iodotyrosines are also quantitated in this method, so that increased levels of these substances, either in disease or after use of drugs, contaminate the application of the PBI method. Hypothyroidism and myxedema are characterized by values below 4 μg/100 ml.

Butanol-Extractable Iodine Butanol extraction eliminates inorganic, ingested, and absorbed iodides, but not iodoproteins. Discrepancies between the PBI and BEI levels are useful in estimating levels of iodoproteins in the presence of biosynthetic defects in the thyroid. Development of methods for T_3 and T_4 measurements by radioimmunoassay render the PBI and BEI methods obsolete, except in the situations cited above.

Total Thyroxine Iodine Thyroid hormone is separated by column chromatography, and quantitation of the iodine content gives a value for T_4 iodine by column. This method provides more reliable data than the previously described procedures for thyroid iodine.

Serum Thyroxine Radioimmunoassay or competitive protein binding (CPB) methods for total thyroxin are not dependent on quantitation of iodine levels in the hormones and are free of contamination by exogenous iodinated materials. Normal values range from 5–13 μg/100 ml.

Serum "Free" Thyroxine Serum "free" thyroxine is determined after a dialysis procedure, after which the CPB method is applied. This is the most sensitive and accurate method of quantitating the active levels of T_4 in the serum.

Free Thyroxin Index A method of calculating a free thyroxine index employs the total T_4 level or PBI and the assessment of the amount of binding proteins after this formula:

$$T_4 \text{ index} = \text{total } T_4 \times \text{resin } T_3 \text{ uptake}/30$$

Normal values range from 5–13 μg/100 ml. If the PBI is employed:

$$\text{thyroid index} = \text{PBI} \times \text{resin } T_3 \text{ uptake}/30$$

Normal values range from 4.2–7.8 μg/100 ml.

Serum Triiodothyronine Levels Serum triiodothyronine levels (T_3) by radioimmunoassay have been devised by Hollander et al. (1972). Circulating levels in normal subjects range from 60–220 ng/100 ml. Hyperthyroidism is associated with values considerably in excess of 220 ng/100 ml, and such high values may antedate elevations in the other parameters of estimating thyroid gland function.

Thyroid Hormone Binding by Serum Proteins as Index of Thyroid Function
Resin T₃-Uptake

A tracer amount of ^{131}I labeled T_3 is added to serum containing an insoluble anion exchange resin or charcoal, and the amount of labeled T_3 retained in the insoluble phase represents the resin T_3 uptake (fig. 9.3). This value is a measure of the reserve binding capacity in the serum. Increased thyroid hormone in the serum leads to a greater saturation of the binding capacity, so that the insoluble resin takes up more of the labeled T_3, *i.e.*, an increased resin T_3 uptake is found in hyperthyroidism. In hypothyroidism, decreased levels of thyroid hormones leave a larger amount of unsaturated binding sites, hence, the labeled T_3 is picked up by these sites instead of onto the insoluble resin. Hence, there is a decreased resin T_3 uptake in hypothyroidism.

Several factors alter the thyroid-binding capacity of the serum proteins. Pregnancy, or estrogen administration, induce increased levels of TBG, thus resin T_3 uptake is low in these states, despite the absence of thyroid disease.

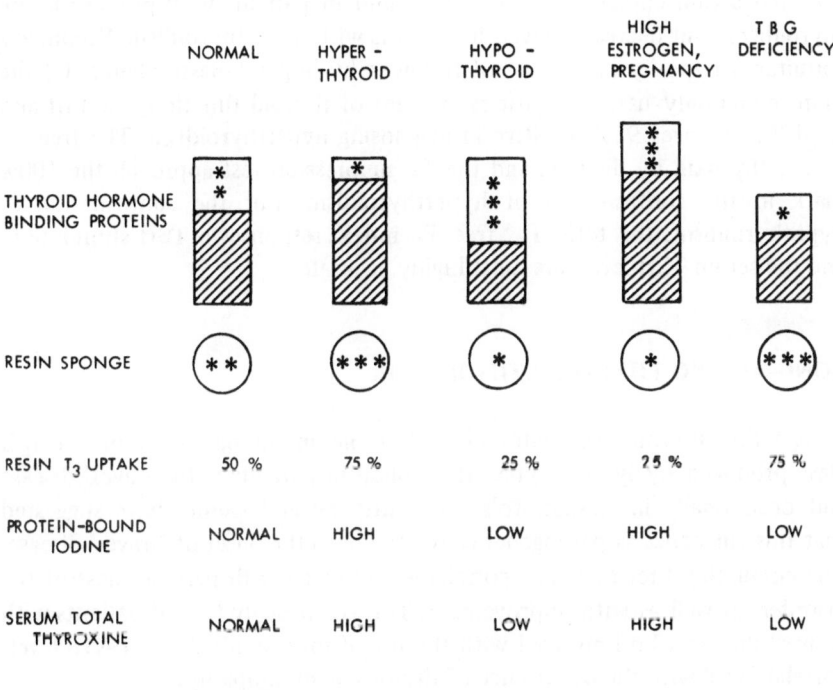

	NORMAL	HYPER-THYROID	HYPO-THYROID	HIGH ESTROGEN, PREGNANCY	TBG DEFICIENCY
RESIN T₃ UPTAKE	50 %	75 %	25 %	? 5 %	75 %
PROTEIN-BOUND IODINE	NORMAL	HIGH	LOW	HIGH	LOW
SERUM TOTAL THYROXINE	NORMAL	HIGH	LOW	HIGH	LOW

KEY : ▨ THYROID HORMONES BOUND TO BINDING PROTEINS

▭ UNSATURATED BINDING PROTEIN

* ^{131}I LABELLED T_3

Figure 9.3.   Principles of the resin uptake of ^{131}IT_3 uptake test (RU'T₃).

Tests Based on Metabolic Effects of Thyroid Hormones

Clinical procedures to measure biologic activity of its hormones include: basal metabolic rate (BMR); Achilles tendon reflex time; and miscellaneous tests.

Basal Metabolic Rate The basal metabolic rate varies directly with the level of thyroid function and, in euthyroidism, ranges between −10 to +10% of normal. Myxedematous patients exhibit a value of below −30%, while hyperthyroid subjects may show values of +25 to +75%. Despite its usefulness, this test is not widely employed now. Several technical problems, including leaks in the metabolometer, lack of patient cooperation, the emotional state of the patient, as well as nonthyroidal illnesses, may alter the basal metabolism rate.

Achilles Tendon Reflex Measurement The Achilles tendon reflex measurement is based on the observation that there is a significant delay in the relaxation phase of the deep tendon reflexes. The procedure is recommended only to provide secondary confirmation of hypothyroidism.

Miscellaneous Tests Miscellaneous tests include the measurement of serum cholesterol which is inversely related to the level of primary function. Elevated serum cholesterol levels are found in patients with primary hypothyroidism, and decreased levels in patients with hyperthyroidism. Secondary (pituitary) hypothyroidism is not followed by hypercholesterolemia. Of the more commonly used tests for assessment of thyroid function, the PBI and total T_4 are over 95% sensitive in diagnosing hyperthyroidism. The free T_4 index, thyroxin by dialysis, and the T_3 suppression test approach the 100% mark in the confirmation of hyperthyroidism. For the confirmation of hypothyroidism, the total T_4, free T_4 index, response to TSH stimulation, and the serum TSH levels are most highly accurate.

LONG-ACTING THYROID STIMULATOR

Long-acting thyroid stimulator (LATS) is an immunoglobulin of the IgG class produced by lymphocytes. It is found in patients with Graves' disease and occasionally in Hashimoto's thyroiditis. Several studies have suggested that this substance is pathogenetically related to the onset of Graves' disease. The circulating titer of LATS correlates quite well with pervasiveness of the disorder, as well as with improvement. This is especially true of patients with Graves' disease who improved with the use of thionamide drugs. LATS levels correlate well with the occurrence of thyrotoxic dermopathy.

Experimental studies reveal an effect of LATS on release of membrane adenyl cyclase in the thyroid quite similar to the influence of TSH. There has been strong evidence that LATS is responsible for the onset of neonatal thyrotoxicosis in babies of Graves' disease mothers. However, a recent report showed that this is not necessarily true. There are data that Graves' disease does not comply with the postulates required for an autoimmunity disorder. The current concept now is that LATS is not the sole cause of Graves' disease, but it plays a major contributory role in its pathogenesis.

HYPERTHYROIDISM

Hyperthyroidism refers to the multisystem disorders arising from increased circulating levels of thyroid hormones, thyroxine (T_4), and triiodothyronine (T_3), the iodothyronines. Etiology of the various types of hyperthyroidism are presented in figure 9.4.

Clinical Manifestations of Hyperthyroidism

The clinical manifestations observed in patients with hyperthyroidism, regardless of type of etiology, are presented in table 9.1. Many of these features are due to the interaction of thyroid hormones and catecholamines, as there is synergism in many of their actions. Features unique to specific types of hyperthyroidism are considered below.

Special Manifestations of Different Forms of Hyperthyroidism

Atypical patterns of hyperthyroidism include the following.

Hypertriodothyroninemia or T_3-Toxicosis This disorder has been described by Hollander et al. (1972) and others. It has undoubtedly been more prevalent than previously recognized. In the past, the diagnosis was suspected in patients who exhibited all the features of hyperthyroidism, lacking laboratory confirmation by standard methods but demonstrating nonsuppressibility of thyroid RAI uptake by exogenous T_3. With new methodology, the diagnosis is made more readily with these criteria.

The criteria for diagnosis of T_3-toxicosis are: (1) clinical picture of hyperthyroidism and hypermetabolism; (2) normal levels of PBI and total T_4; (3) normal levels of free T_4; (4) normal or slight to moderate increase in epithyroid RAI uptake which is not suppressible by the T_3 suppression test (triiodothyronine 25 μg 3 times daily for 7–10 days); (5) an increased total T_3 level (normal level = 80–220 ng/100 ml); and (6) demonstration of pituitary thyrotropic suppression by absent TSH levels or by lack of pituitary response to TRF.

In addition to the full-fledged T_3-toxicosis pattern, certain variants have been described. These include hyperthyroninemia as a premonitory manifestation of thyrotoxicosis (Hollander et al., 1971), T_3 elevation during antithyroid drug therapy for hyperthyroidism, T_3 elevation as an early manifesta-

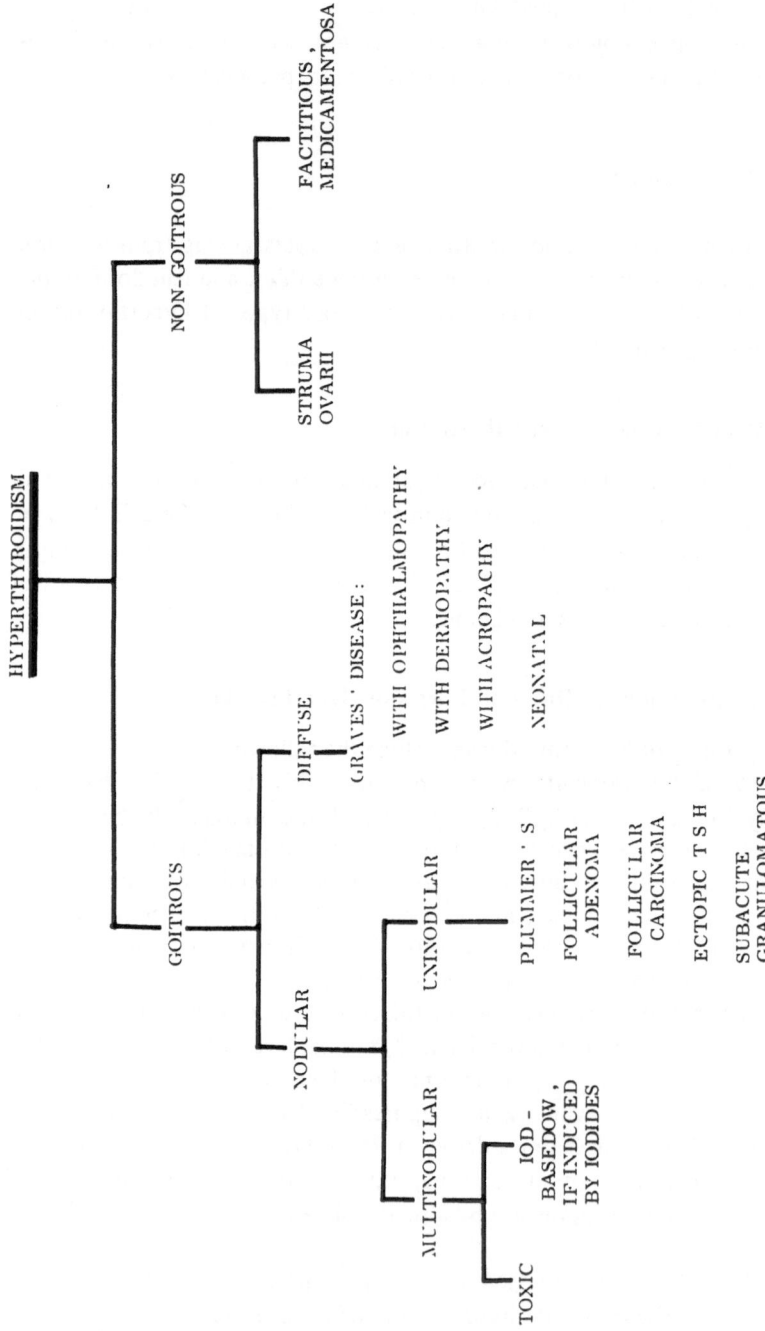

Figure 9.4. Classification of hyperthyroidism. Some authorities include multinodular hyperthyroidism under the term Plummer's disease.

Table 9.1. Clinical Manifestations in Patients with Hyperthyroidism

I. Symptoms of hyperthyroidism
  A. Referrable to enhanced catecholamine effects (nervousness; tremors; palpitations; rapid heart rate; increased perspiration; heat intolerance)
  B. Referrable to hypermetabolism (mild hyperpyrexia; increased appetite and hyperphagia; weight loss usually, but weight gain may occur as an early manifestation)
  C. Increased autonomic activity (diarrhea due to decreased transit time)
  D. Miscellaneous (myopathy with muscle weakness; periodic paralysis; dyspnea due to weakness of respiratory muscles; personality changes; psychosis; criminal behavior; hypermentation; restlessness; hair loss; symptoms of high output failure; lid retraction with staring; opthalmopathy)
II. Clinical signs in hyperthyroidism
  A. Skin and appendages (smooth pink elbows; soft, smooth, velvety skin texture; fine hair structure; palmar erythema; onycholysis; increased sweating; vitiligo, or hyperpigmentation)
  B. Cardiovascular and respiratory systems (increased pulse pressure due to increased systolic blood pressure; increased pulse rate; increased cardiac stroke volume; dilated peripheral vascular bed; high output cardiac failure, depending on severity, atrial fibrillation (10–15%); decreased pulmonary compliance; weakness in respiratory muscles leading to dyspnea)
  C. Gastrointestinal system (diarrhea and/or hyperdefecation; hypochlorhydria (30% have antibodies to parietal cells); hepatocellular dysfunction; lipid infiltration; increased clearance of various substrates; hypoalbuminemia may be due to hepatocellular disease or to hypercatabolism)
  D. Nervous system (hyperkinesis; tremors, increased energy followed by fatigability; hyperreflexia followed by hypo- or areflexia if myopathy becomes severe)
  E. Ocular system (ophthalmopathy in Graves' disease, variable and including unilateral or bilateral exophthalmos; proptosis; edema of the eyelids; conjunctival injection; chemosis; ophthalmoplegia due to edema of extra occular muscles; lid retraction (Dalrymple's sign); lid lag (von Graefe's sign); globe lag; loss of sight from optic nerve involvement)
  F. Locomotor system (proximal muscle weakness, may be unable to climb stairs because of thigh muscle weakness; periodic paralysis, may be associated with hypokalemia, seen especially in Orientals)
  G. Reproductive system (delayed sexual maturation if hyperthyroidism starts early in life; accelerated skeletal growth; increased libido in both sexes; an ovulatory menstrual cycle; oligomenorrhea, or amenorrhea)
  H. Renal system (increased renal blood flow and glomerular filtration rate (GFR); increased tubular reabsorption and secretion)
  I. Hematopoietic system (occasionally erythrocytosis, but anemia may also occur; relative lymphocytosis and granulocytopenia)
  J. Pituitary and adrenocortical function (exaggeration of circadian variation of plasma cortisol; accelerated disappearance of cortisol from blood stream; increased conversion of cortisol to cortisone, the latter being biologically less active; increased reduction of the Δ^4, 3-ketone structure of ring A, thus inactivating the biologic activity, attenuated growth hormone response to insulin)

tion of recurrent hyperthyroidism, *e.g.,* following inadequate thionamide drug therapy or after inadequate ^{131}I therapy, and T_3 elevation in iodine deficiency. There are data suggesting that the T_3 levels in T_3-toxicosis may vary according to the type of gland involvement, viz., in diffuse toxic goiter the levels will be higher than in uninodular and multinodular toxic goiter.

Hyperthyroidism without Evident Goiter Werner and Ingbar (1971) have described hyperthyroidism without palpably enlarged goiter in 1–3% of hyperthyroid patients.

Hyperthyroidism without Overt Hypermetabolism Hyperthyroidism without overt hypermetabolism was established by basal metabolic rate values which were within normal ranges, but PBI and RAI uptake were elevated. Both these parameters reverted to normal after therapy.

Euthyroid Graves' Disease with Ocular Changes Ophthalmopathy has been described in overtly euthyroid patients who, nevertheless, had some evidence of autonomous thyroid activity.

Apathetic Hyperthyroidism Apathetic hyperthyroidism describes the clinical state of elderly patients with laboratory evidence of hyperthyroidism but overtly lacking many of the other clinical manifestations of hyperthyroidism except for the cardiovascular components. These patients are prone to progress rapidly into thyroid storm and die suddenly if the diagnosis is not made and the disorder is not treated.

Natural Course of Hyperthyroidism

This discussion refers more specifically to diffuse toxic goiter, but may, in some considerations, apply also to nodular toxic goiter. Etiology of these disorders is not known despite the preferred relationship between LATS and Graves' disease. Many predisposing factors have been described, including genetic susceptibility, familial tendency, and previous nutritional history. Precipitating factors include physical or emotional trauma, stress, illness, accident, pregnancy, puberty, and labor, among others.

There are old data which indicate that significant numbers of patients may undergo spontaneous remission (Means, 1948). The reason for these remissions is not clear either. It is not possible now to design a study to determine the natural course of this disorder. Older statistics indicate that about 15–20% of patients died during the active phase of thyrotoxicosis (presumably of the disorder) if not treated (Means, 1948). Spontaneous remission in 26–50% of untreated patients and a 15–30% rate of improvement have been described (Sattler, 1952).

It is now becoming apparent that, in a large number of patients, Graves' disease evolves first into euthyroidism followed by hypothyroidism. Follow-up of patients treated with high dose ^{131}I revealed 20% become hypothyroid within 1 yr of therapy, with an additional 3%/yr thereafter. When a low dose of ^{131}I was employed, it became apparent that the rate of development of hypothyroidism was slowed for the first 1–3 yr, but the subsequent course was similar to those treated with the higher doses of radiation. Careful followup of patients treated by surgery revealed a similar evolution into hypothyroidism. The above data suggest that the natural course of hyperthyroidism in the patient who survives the acute phase includes a period of remission followed by hypothyroidism (fig. 9.5).

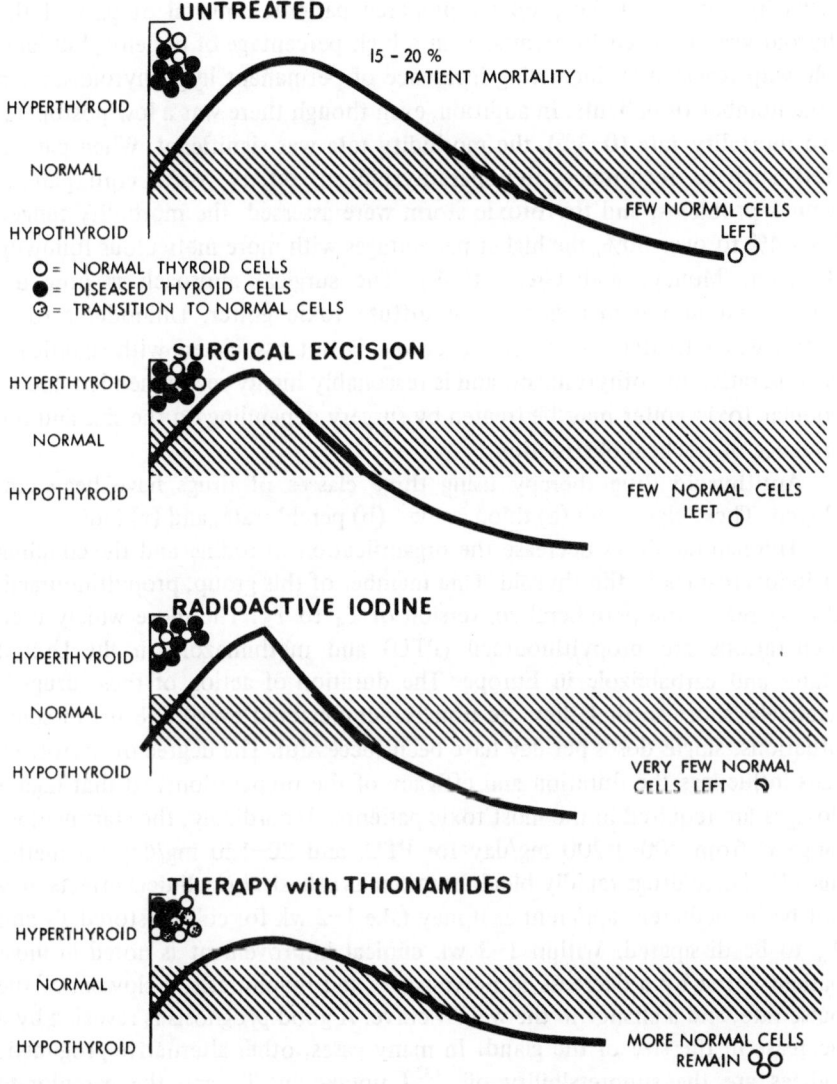

Figure 9.5. Natural history of diffuse toxic goiter and effects of different methods of management. It is shown that radioiodine therapy and surgical excision remove a number of euthyroid cells from the total thyroidal cell pool. It is suggested that the thionanide drugs may alter some hyperthyroid cells to the euthyroid state, hence, potentially altering the natural progression toward hypothyroidism.

Treatment of Hyperthyroidism

Management will depend on the type of hyperthyroidism. Major consideration will be given to the management of diffuse toxic goiter, but multinodular
and uninodular toxic goiters will also be considered.

Three therapeutic measures are available: (1) surgery; (2) antithyroid
drugs; and (3) radioiodine therapy.

Surgery has been extensively employed in the management of all types of
hyperthyroidism. In the properly prepared patient, removal of part of the
thyroid was followed by remission in a high percentage of patients, but later
followup revealed an increasing incidence of permanent hypothyroidism in a
large number of patients. In addition, even though there was a low postoperative mortality rate (0–3%), the morbidity rate was significant. When parameters such as recurrence, hypoparathyroidism, tetany, vocal cord paresis,
wound problems, and thyrotoxic storm were assessed, the morbidity ranged
from 4% to over 30%, the higher percentages with more meticulous followup
(Rawson, Money, and Greif, 1969). The surgical approach is now de-
emphasized in the management of diffuse toxic goiter. Uninodular toxic
goiter, when treated by surgical excision, is not associated with significant
postoperative hypothyroidism, and is reasonably highly recommended. Multinodular toxic goiter may be treated by surgery depending on the size and the
presence of tracheal obstruction.

Antithyroid drug therapy using three classes of drugs have been employed. These classes are (a) thionamides, (b) perchlorate, and (c) iodine.

Thionamide drugs decrease the organification of iodine and the coupling
of iodotyrosines in the thyroid. One member of this group, propylthiouracil,
also decreases the peripheral conversion of T_4 to T_3. The more widely used
preparations are propylthiouracil (PTU) and methimazole in the United
States and carbamizole in Europe. The duration of action of these drugs is
relatively short so that they are usually administered every 6–8 hr. In some
situations, single doses per day have been successful. The degree of thyrotoxi-
cans influences the duration and efficacy of the preparations, so that higher
dosages are required in the most toxic patients. Accordingly, the starting dose
range is from 200–1,200 mg/day for PTU, and 20–120 mg/day for methimazole. These drugs rapidly block hormone synthesis, but clinical effects may
not be immediately apparent as it may take 1–2 wk for colloid-stored T_4 and
T_3 to be dissipated. Within 1–3 wk clinical improvement is noted in most
patients, first by a decrease in nervousness and diaphoresis, a slowing of the
pulse rate, and a change in the weight curve. A good prognosis is revealed by a
decrease in the size of the gland. In many cases, other alternative prognostic
indices are the suppressibility of ^{131}I uptake by T_3 and the perchlorate
washout test. Depending on the response, it is recommended that the patient
be committed to 6–12 mo of the first course of therapy. Dosage of drugs is
decreased soon after there is evidence of improvement, or may be increased if

there is no improvement within 2–3 wk. An enlargement of the gland, after initial decrease in size, indicates over treatment and induction of hypothyroidism. This may be confirmed by a plasma TSH level. This is not a frequent problem with reasonably careful followup. Cutaneous allergies and agranulocytosis may occur in a few patients on these drugs. The incidence of such problems is from 0.7–3.0%. Occasional leukocyte counts may be made, but they are not necessarily of predictive value. The patient should be cautioned to stop the drug if an unexplained sore throat or rash should appear after institution of the medication. In that event, an alternative drug is tried. Worldwide statistics indicate a 40–60% permanent remission rate with one course (6–18 mo) of therapy. A secondary course of therapy is followed by a similar remission rate. Most authorities recommend an alternative method of management after failure with two courses. Tertiary courses have occasionally been successful, however. The low incidence of permanent hypothyroidism following medical therapy suggests that the natural history may well be altered by this method. This form of therapy is also recommended in pediatric hyperthyroidism, although some patients have been treated with [131] I. Short-term medical therapy with thionamides is often used for preoperative preparation, with iodine added for several days prior to surgery. A widely used preparatory method prior to surgery is the use of propranolol to suppress the catecholamine-iodothyronine synergism.

Perchlorate prevents iodide uptake by thyroid, and this method has been used therapeutically. Because of the occurrence of aplastic anemia following its use, the drug is now restricted.

[131] I is quite useful in the management of diffuse toxic goiter and in many cases of multinodular toxic goiter. Extensive use permits statistical evaluation of its efficacy. The heavy dose therapy 14,000 rads is followed by reasonably prompt remission of the disorder (3–4 mo), but a 20% occurrence of permanent hypothyroidism is noted within 1 yr, increasing roughly 5–6%/yr thereafter. Conventional dose thereapy (7,000 rads) also produces reasonably rapid remission, but a 10–15% incidence of hyperthyroidism within 1 yr and 3% each succeeding year has been observed. One-half of the conventional dose (3,500 rads) is followed by a measurable rate of hypothyroidism also.

A relatively new approach is to palliate the patient with β-adrenergic blocking agents such as propranolol until a spontaneous remission of the process occurs. But this method does not alter the long-term occurrence of hypothyroidism.

Thyrotoxic Storm

Thyrotoxic storm (thyroid storm) represents an exaggerated phase of thyrotoxicosis in which the etiology of the acute complication is unknown. It has frequently been precipitated by surgery and by several medical stresses, *e.g.*, diabetic ketoacidosis, fright, toxemia of pregnancy, parturition. Withdrawal from iodine therapy has also been suggested as a precipitating cause. The mechanism is ascribed to suppressed hormone release while the patient is on iodine, with rapid release of hormone from an iodine-enriched gland on sudden withdrawal of the drug. Radioiodine therapy, by causing postradiation thyroiditis, may also precipitate this clinical emergency. Ether anesthesia is associated with increased dissociation of T_4 from tissue stores and may precipitate this disorder. Other factors include alterations in differential protein binding of T_3 and T_4.

Thyrotoxic storm is seen mainly in diffuse toxic goiter, but has occasionally arisen in multinodular toxic goiter. It is usually of abrupt onset, and hyperpyrexia is a *sine qua non* of the diagnosis. The fever may reach lethal levels within 1–2 days. The patient usually has most of the stigmata of thyrotoxicosis. Atrial fibrillation or other tachyarrhythmias may be present, and acute pulmonary edema or congestive heart failure may supervene. Systolic hypertension, as in uncomplicated hyperthyroidism, may later change to hypotension and shock. The usual central nervous system manifestations of hyperthyroidism may be replaced by stupor or coma. Diarrhea may be a major manifestation.

Differential diagnosis to rule out superimposed problems is important because therapy for the storm and for hyperthyroidism is similar, while intercurrent problems may require special therapy. Laboratory data are not of any additional help over and above the diagnosis of hyperthyroidism. Specific treatment goals are to stop the increased synthesis and secretion of T_4 and T_3, to suppress the iodothyronine-catecholamine target effects, to treat the precipitating illness, and to support body defense mechanisms, *e.g.*, to treat congestive failure, atrial fibrillation, and shock if they occur.

Antithyroid drugs should be instituted first to achieve the first goal above. PTU in the amount of 1,200–1,500 mg/day (or tapazol in the amount of 120–150 mg) given orally, or crushed and given by nasogastric tube if necessary, should be instituted. PTU is probably better, as it depresses conversion of T_4 to T_3 in the periphery, whereas methimazole does not. Iodide therapy is employed to decrease the release of T_4 and T_3 from the gland. Lugol's iodine (30 drops/day orally) or sodium iodide (1–2 g by slow intravenous drip) are recommended. Antithyroid drugs should precede use of iodine, as they will block the organification and coupling of iodine in the gland. Blockage of the iodothyronine-catecholamine interaction requires the use of drugs which deplete catecholamines or prevent their action. These drugs are reserpine, guanethidine, and propranolol. Reserpine up to 2.5 mg intravenously 4–6 times/day is recommended because of its depressant effect, but should be avoided in shock. Guanethidine (50–150 g/day) is also useful for this treatment but must be avoided in patients in shock. Propranolol, a β-adrenergic blocker, may be administered parenterally 1–2 mg intravenously under electrocardiogram control; this dosage is repeatable in 2 min. Treatment of the precipitating illness requires a vigorous search for a coexistent or precipitating disorder, such as febrile, inflammatory, or infectious disease, and institution of the appropriate therapy. Supportive management of the physiologic or biochemical aberrations may occur, so that for congestive heart failure, the use of digitalis preparations (and diuretics) is required. Measures for alleviation of hyperpyrexia, including replenishment of fluids if dehydration is a factor or glucose infusion for caloric replacement, are necessary. Some may elect to use glucocorticoids at a dose range of 100–300 mg Solu-Cortef daily. The rationale for this therapy may be that the effective cortisol levels are lower because of the activation of 11-dehydrogenation of cortisol (with formation of cortisone, biologically less active) by excess thyroid hormones. With this method of management most patients should show improvement within 24–36 hr with complete recovery from this complication within 5 days. Further therapy of hyperthyroidism was discussed in another section.

Treatment of Eye Changes in Graves' Disease

The fullness, lacrimation, and opthalmoplegia in this disorder may be aided by sleeping with the head elevated, as many of these changes are due to edematous changes. Corneal injury may be prevented by use of glasses and lubricant drops or ophthalmic ointments, and local therapy with guanethidine drops to produce a Horner's syndrome has occasionally been helpful. In severe proptosis, decompression measures may become necessary.

Because of the possibility that surgical or ^{131}I therapy for hyperthyroidism may be associated with exacerbation of the eye changes, many physicians prefer therapy with antithyroid drugs. Despite the method of therapy, however, exophthalmos may progress. Systemic drug therapy as described below has been attempted with some degree of success. (1) Prednisone therapy (100–125 mg daily) has been used to suppress the muscle and visual impairment. Therapy in severe cases is continued for 6–8 mo. Many untoward effects of steroid therapy may occur in this period of time. Milder degrees of eye involvement have been treated with smaller doses of steroids. Replacement of potassium chloride and other protective measures used should be employed when heavy doses are given. (2) Diuretic agents have been tried, but are only mildly successful. (3) X-ray therapy to the pituitary has been tried without marked success. (4) X-ray therapy to the retrobulbar areas has met with some measures of success.

Surgical decompression measures are required when the lids are so tense and edematous that lid adhesions cannot be performed. Such measures protect the globe by relieving pressure within the orbit.

Treatment of Nodular Toxic Goiter

The two major forms of goitrous hyperthyroidism (fig. 9-1) differ in pathogenesis and course. The multinodular goiter which may become hyperactive
usually starts as a nontoxic goiter with structural features which suggest
different degrees of activity in various parts of the gland; some areas showing
hyperplasia and evidence of autonomous control. There are data suggesting an
excessive production of T_3, the biologically more active iodothyronine. The
disorder is more prevalent in patients over 50 yr who have had a nontoxic
multinodular gland for years. The cardiovascular manifestations, including
atrial fibrillation or tachycardia (often resistant to digitalis), are prominent.
Muscle wasting and weakness are often found. The preferred treatment in
patients with this disorder is radioactive iodine in conventional doses. But
many of these patients may require preliminary control with the thionamide
drugs, the β-adrenergic blocking agents, or both.

Uninodular toxic goiter (toxic adenoma) is less common than the two
other forms of goitrous hyperthyroidism. The toxic adenoma is a true
follicular adenoma which is autonomous and not responsive to the hypothalamic-pituitary axis. The goiter is palpable as a single nodule which is also
detected by the discrete increased radioiodine uptake. The surrounding thyroid tissue exhibits suppressed uptake due to the decreased TSH levels
secondary to elevated iodothyronine levels. This disorder is most often seen
in patients in their thirties or forties. The clinical manifestations are usually
milder than in Graves' disease, with the cardiovascular manifestations quite
prominent. Infiltrative ophthalmopathy is not usually found.

Surgical ablative therapy is the recommended therapy, especially if the
contiguous thyroid function is suppressed. Preparative therapy may involve
the use of propranolol or, as in the pregnant thyrotoxic patient, of thionamides. The adenoma responds well to radioiodine therapy also, but this
therapy is followed by the presence of a "cold" nodule, the nature of which
may raise questions at some subsequent time.

Thyrotoxicosis in Pregnancy

Hyperthyroidism complicates pregnancy in 0.047–0.1% of patients. Despite
alterations in menstrual cycle by hyperthyroidism, such patients may become
pregnant. It has been suggested, and discounted, that pregnancy may be a
precipitating factor in the pathogenesis of hyperthyroidism. Many features of
pregnancy imitate hyperthyroidism, for example, skin texture, slight systolic
hypertension, a slight temperature rise, and often an enlargement in the
thyroid gland. However, if true hyperthyroidism is present, there are usually
several additional features. Laboratory diagnosis is relatively simple if the
alterations in TBG induced by pregnancy (via estrogens) are kept in mind.

Accordingly, in the pregnant state, the PBI and total T_4 are elevated, while the resin uptake of T_3 is depressed. Calculation of the thyroid index from these data will confirm euthyroidism. Hyperthyroidism superimposed in pregnancy is associated with higher levels of PBI and total T_4, and the RU T_3 will be increased so that the calculated thyroid index will be unquestionably in the hyperthyroid range (see section on laboratory methods). Determination of a free T_4 by dialysis will confirm the diagnosis, but this is unnecessary under most conditions. It should be emphasized that diagnostic thyroid ^{131}I uptake is not recommended in pregnancy, because of potential hazard to the fetal thyroid.

Treatment of Hyperthyroidism in Pregnancy

Therapeutic abortions are not needed for conventional hyperthyroidism, as medical therapy of the hypermetabolic state is available. The goals of management are to achieve euthyroidism before time of delivery in order to avoid thyroid storm which may be precipitated by labor and delivery, and to achieve euthyroidism by measures which are not harmful to mother or baby. The two available safe methods applicable in pregnancy are surgery and antithyroid drugs. The use of iodine is absolutely contraindicated because the ingested iodine, on reaching the fetal thyroid, will suppress thyroid hormone release by the intrathyroidal iodide autoregulation mechanism. Negative feedback regulation will precipitate an increased release of TSH, which will induce a goiter. Radioiodine therapy is contraindicated, as stated above. Surgery is not recommended in the first or third trimesters, and is considered only in the second trimester. By this time, the patient should be essentially euthyroid if precipitation of thyroid storm and all its hazards are to be avoided. It is, therefore, essential that the patient be given a course of antithyroid drugs to achieve euthyroidism by the second trimester. Since the natural outcome of a given hyperthyroid gland is not predictable, as indeed there may well be spontaneous remissions, some thought should be given to continuing antithyroid drugs and avoid ablative surgery.

Of the antithyroid drugs, the thionamides commonly employed block the organic binding of iodine and the coupling of iodotyrosines in the thyroid. In addition, propylthiouracil blocks the conversion of T_4 to the more active T_3. Management of the pregnant patient with antithyroid drugs requires awareness that these drugs cross the placental barrier and will affect the fetal thyroid and thyroid-pituitary axis. This effect is directly correlated with the dosage of the drugs used. The required dosage is also related to the degree of thyrotoxicosis in the mother, as the biologic decay of the drugs will be enhanced by increased hypermetabolism. It is, therefore, necessary to employ dosages sufficient to suppress maternal thyroid overactivity, while not sufficient to significantly affect fetal hormonogenesis and TSH release. Propylthiouracil (600 mg/day) or tapazol (60 mg/day) may be employed in early pregnancy. These doses are given as one-fourth every 6 hr or one-third every 8 hr. With this dosage, it is possible in most patients to achieve euthyroidism before the start of the third trimester, at which time a considerably lower dose may be used. Recent reports suggest that propranolol may be safely used throughout pregnancy palliatively in the hope of eventual remission or definitive management later. Some authorities have used thyroid extract or thyroxin concurrently in order to suppress fetal TSH overproduction in the event of significant antithyroid drug effect on the fetal thyroid. This concept may be fallacious in part, as the high TBG levels in the maternal circulation may effectively deter much transfer of T_4 to the fetal compartment. It might be more useful to use T_3 supplements because of their weaker affinity for TBG. We have rarely added thyroid hormone supplements in the management of our thyrotoxic pregnant patients. Previous surveys have shown the occasional occurrence of fetal goiters following the maternal use of antithyroid drugs, but these occurred when larger doses were employed and, occasionally, when iodides were added to the regimen.

HYPOTHYROIDISM

Hypothyroidism is due to a deficiency of thyroid hormones (T_4 and/or T_3), with resulting decrease or absence of the peripheral effects of the hormones. The hypothyroid states are classified in the list that follows. Regardless of the basis of the deficiency of the iodothyronine hormones, there are several features common to all hypothyroid states. Special features relative either to age of onset or to specific types of disorders are discussed in a subsequent section. The symptoms of hypothyroidism are referrable to several organ systems. Decreased cellular metabolism and oxygen consumption are the probable bases for apathy, lethargy, somnolence, cold intolerance, bradycardia, and moderate weight gain. Constipation is occasionally sufficiently severe to lead to fecal impaction. Muscle cramps may occur with or without activity. Dyspnea due to decreased breathing capacity and alveolar hypoventilation may occur. Many patients may experience hair loss and loss of the lateral eyebrows. Decreased libido has been described in hypothyroid patients of both sexes, and impotence may occur in males. Hypermenorrhea is probably secondary to endometrial hyperplasia secondary to prolonged estrogen effect due to abnormal feedback regulation of the pituitary-ovarian axis (Chapter 5). The clinical signs of hypothyroidism are:

1. Skin and appendages (dermal glycoprotein deposition (myxedema) with nonpitting puffiness especially around eyes and hands; decreased sweating; coarse, brittle hair (especially on back and extremities in children); follicular hyperkeratosis; malar flush, and yellowish discoloration in other areas)

2. Cardiovascular system (bradycardia; decreased stroke volume; decreased

cardiac output; increased vascular resistance; dilated heart with pale flabby myocardium; electrocardiogram may be normal or may show how P, ORS, and T, occasional rightward T vector; increased susceptibility to cardiac glycosides; decreased blood flow)

3. Respiratory system (decreased maximum breathing capacity and alveolar hypoventilation)

4. Gastrointestinal system (delayed dentition in children; broad thick tongue; hypochlorhydria and enlargement of intestinal tract in some patients; delayed absorption of carbohydrates, fats, proteins, vitamins, and minerals; distention, abdominal pain, and vomiting leading to paralytic ileus; decreased hepatic clearance of several substrates)

5. Nervous system (slowing of intellectual function; slow and clumsy movements; occasional cerebellar ataxia; diminished deep tendon reflexes; dysarthria, carpal tunnel syndrome; myxedematous dementia; cretinous deafness, and deaf mutism in Pendred's syndrome)

6. Locomotor system (decreased growth and bone maturation; decreased bone turnover)

7. Reproductive system (menorrhagia; metrorrhagia; occasional amenorrhea; male patients on rare occasions may have oligospermia or normal sperm counts with low inability percentage)

8. Renal system (decreased glomerular filtration rate (GFR); decreased renal blood flow; tubular dysfunction manifested by decreased resorptive and secretory maximal capacities; decreased water diuresis)

9. Hematopoietic system (decreased red cell mass with normocytic normochromic anemia; presumably decreased O_2 dissociation prevents erythropoietin release; occasionally pernicious anemia may be secondary to achlorhydria and lack of intrinsic factor production in the gastric mucosa in hypothyroidism; a malabsorption of B_{12} intrinsic factor complex due to ileal mucosal defect has been noted occasionally; clotting factors VIII and IX are decreased)

10. Pituitary-adrenocortical-axis function (decreased conversion of cortisol to cortisone; decreased urinary 17-OHCS and 17-KS; decreased plasma cortisol levels with attenuated circadian rhythmicity)

Laboratory Diagnosis of Hypothyroidism

The rationales and accuracy of the various laboratory tests of thyroid function were discussed previously. Differential diagnosis of these disorders by laboratory procedures is presented in table 9.2.

Treatment of Hypothyroidism

The goal of therapy is to replace thyroid hormones to achieve euthyroid levels. The clinical end points are well-being of the patient, skin structure,

Table 9.2. Classification of Hypothyroid States and Appropriate Laboratory Data

Disorder	RAI uptake	RAI after TSH	Perchlorate washout	TSH levels	TRH stimulation	Special tests
Goitrous defects in:						
Iodide trapping	↓	↓	Discharged	↑	Not needed	Low MIT and DIT
Organification	↑	↑	Discharged	↑	Not needed	Measure iodotyrosines
Coupling	↑	↑	N[a]	↑	Not needed	Measure iodotyrosines
Deiodinase	↑		N	↑	Not needed	Separation of iodoproteins
Abnormal iodoprotein		↑	N	↑	Not needed	
Deaf mutism with end-organ resistance			N	↑	Not needed	
Endemic cretinism	↓	↓	N	↑	Not needed	
Goitrogen Rx	N	N	N or discharged	↑	Not needed	
Nongoitrous defects in:						
Idiopathic myxedema	↓	↓	Not needed	↑	Not needed	
Congenital athyreosis	↓	↓	Not needed	↑	Not needed	
Thyroid destruction	↓	↑	Not needed	↑	Not needed	
TSH deficiency	↓	↑	Not needed	↓, N	No change	
Panhypopituitarism	↓	↑	Not needed	↓, N	No change	
Hypothalamic hypothyroidism	↓	↑	Not needed	↓, N	↑	

pulse rate, as well as improvement in several of the parameters affected by the disorder. Three thyroid preparations are available for therapeutic use: desiccated thyroid extract, 1-thyroxine, and triiodothyronine. In all cases of hypothyroidism, full replacement doses of one of these preparations is recommended. Conditions which contraindicate full replacement dosages are arteriosclerotic heart disease with angina pectoris and myxedema-induced heart disease.

The average full replacement doses are: 60–120 mg of thyroid extract, 0.1–0.2 mg of 1-thyroxin, and 25–50 μg of triiodothyronine, with the dose chosen given once daily. T_3 has a faster onset of action and its effect is more rapidly dissipated and, because of this property, it is especially useful in elderly patients with cardiovascular disorders listed above. Such patients are given suboptimal doses such as 5–10 μg of T_3, 0.05 mg of T_4, or 15 mg desiccated thyroid daily for 2 wk or more, and observed for any manifestations of worsened heart disease. The dosage is gradually increased to the closest to full replacement dose tolerable. The replacement program in myxedema coma is described separately. The best current method of gauging adequacy of replacement therapy in primary hypothyroidism is the measurement of plasma TSH levels. Euthyroidism is reflected by TSH values of 0–10 μU/ml.

Secondary hypothyroidism may be due to panhypopituitarism or isolated TSH deficiency. If panhypopituitarism is also present, then the manifestations include those of deficiencies of the various tropic hormones and of growth hormone. Isolated TSH deficiency as a cause of hypothyroidism exhibits some clinical features different from primary hypothyroidism, viz., the skin changes are less noticeable, plasma TSH is not elevated, a TSH stimulation test shows good response, and TSH levels do not increase after TRH injection.

Myxedema coma describes an emergency clinical state due to severe deficiency of thyroid hormones. Clinical features include cachexia in most patients, lethargy progressing to stupor and coma, hypothermia, hypoventilation and respiratory acidosis, hyponatremia, elevated plasma lactate, hypoglycemia, inappropriate antidiuretic hormone, disturbed cerebral metabolism, and rapid progression to death if not treated. There is no spontaneous remission. It is most often seen in the elderly poor, often in patients treated with ^{131}I in the past, and in patients with an unknown cause of hypothyroidism. The acute state may be precipitated by drugs which depress respiration. If this diagnosis is suspected, the following measures are undertaken. Blood is obtained for T_4, T_3, and TSH levels. Treatment is immediately instituted to replace body pool of thyroid hormones and to manage secondary problems. Infusion of sodium L-thyroxine (100–200 μg) is begun. Alternatively, T_3 may be administered orally (75–100 μg). Procedures are undertaken to ensure a clear airway and maintain adequate ventilation, employing assisted ventilation if necessary. Sedative drugs are contraindicated in these patients. If pressor agents are needed for shock, only small amounts are recommended, lest the synergism with thyroid hormones precipitate arrhythmias. A blanket is employed for warmth, but active warming is contraindicated as vascular collapse and increased O_2 consumption may ensue. Glucocorticoid therapy may occasionally be indicated.

THYROID CANCER

Malignant tumors of the thyroid are rare, with deaths from thyroid cancers constituting 0.35% of all cancer deaths in the United States. The three major types of thyroid cancer are papillary carcinoma, follicular carcinoma, and medullary carcinoma. Papillary carcinoma constitutes about 50% of all thyroid cancers and is most prevalent between the second to fifth decades with a 4:1 female to male preponderance. This type of tumor extends by local lymphatic spread to regional nodes. The prognosis is reasonably good after surgical treatment. Follicular carcinoma constitutues 25% of thyroid cancers, occurring mostly in young adults (with higher incidence in women). The tumor spreads by local extension and the prognosis becomes considerably worse if there are distant metastases. This type of tumor is responsive to TSH and takes up [131] I. Radioiodine therapy is therefore useful in these tumors.

Medullary carcinoma are usually large and hard and may be present in both lobes of the thyroid. This type of tumor constitutes 10% of thyroid cancers. The hormone calcitonin is produced in large amounts by these tumors. There is a high association of this tumor with other endocrine tumors, such as pheochromocytoma (Sipple syndrome) and pancreatic tumors.

REFERENCES

Hollander, C. S., T. Mitsuma, A. J. Kastin, L. Shenkman, M. Blum, and D. G. Anderson. 1971. Hypertriodothyroninemia as premonitory manifestation of thyrotoxicosis. Lancet 2:731–733.
Hollander, C. S., N. Nihei, S. Z. Burday, T. Mitsuma, L. Shenkman, and M. Blum. 1972. Clinical and laboratory observations in cases of triiodothyronine toxicosis confirmed by radioimmunoassay. Lancet 1:609–611.
Ingbar, S. H., and K. A. Woeber. The thyroid gland. In R. H. Williams (ed.), Textbook of Endocrinology, pp. 105–286. W. B. Saunders & Company, Philadelphia.
Means, J. H. 1948. The Thyroid and Its Disease. J. B. Lippincott Company, Philadelphia. p. 292.
Rawson, R. W., W. L. Money, and R. L. Grief. 1969. Diseases of the thyroid. In P. K. Bondy, (ed.), Diseases of Metabolism, pp. 753–826. W. B. Saunders Company, Philadelphia

Sattler, H. 1952. Basedow's Disease. Grune & Stratton, Inc., New York.

Shenkman, L. 1972. Hypothalamic control of anterior pituitary function. Am. J. M. S. 263:433–436.

Tata, J. R. 1964. Basal metabolic rate and thyroid hormones. *In* R. Levine and R. Luft (eds.), Advances in Metabolic Disorders. Vol. 1. pp. 153–190. Acad. Press, New York.

Werner, S. C., and H. Hamilton. 1961. Hyperthyroidism without hypermetabolism. J. A. M. A. 146:450–455.

Werner, S. C., and S. H. Ingbar. 1971. The Thyroid. Harper & Row, Publishers, New York.

10

The Adrenal Cortex

Secretions of the adrenal cortex are intimately involved in several aspects of functions of the reproductive system (Forsham, 1969; Bondy, 1969; Bacchus, 1969; Baxter and Forsham, 1972). The participation includes actions of adrenal hormones on the biologic activity of gonadal hormones on their target organs (*e.g.,* permissive action of cortical hormones on breast development), as well as effects of adrenal androgens and estrogens on sexual characteristics and on feedback regulation of the hypothalamic-pituitary-gonadal axis. Detailed discussion of adrenal physiology and disorders of this gland is, therefore, essential in the field of gynecologic endocrinology.

Adrenal cortical cells are derived from mesodermal elements in close connection with the renal and gonadal anlagen. The morphologic zonation into the zona glomerulosa, zona fasciculata, and zona reticularis has been shown to be of significance in terms of biosynthetic activity, the zona glomerulosa secreting the mineralocorticoid hormone aldosterone, and the inner zones secreting the glucocorticoid hormone cortisol as well as the androgens and estrogens. In the human (and other mammalian) adrenal glands, the cortical cells are supplied by arterial branches which enter sinusoidal circulation in the cortex, eventually draining into a single vein from each gland.

ADRENOCORTICAL SECRETION

Adrenocorticotropic Hormone

Pituitary ACTH stimulates the secretion of the glucocorticoid hormones, cortisol and corticosterone, by the zona fasciculata. Secretion and release of the mineralocorticoid principle aldosterone depend on the renin-angiotensin mechanism. Biosynthetic activities in this zone are dependent on the availability of steroid substrates, which are provided from cholesterol through

ACTH action on the inner zones. ACTH supports growth of adrenal cells by increasing RNA replication.

ACTH release is under the control of the hypothalamus and higher central nervous system centers which influence the hypothalamic corticotropin-releasing factor (CRF). Circulating levels of cortisol regulate ACTH release by a negative feedback mechanism, whereby high levels of cortisol depress release of hypothalamic CRF and, subsequently, of pituitary ACTH. Low levels of cortisol, as in primary adrenal insufficiency, stimulate increased ACTH release by the intact pituitary. Cortisone and aldosterone possess some of the ACTH suppression activity, but the mineralocorticoid, desoxycortico-sterone, which may accumulate in certain biosynthetic defects in the adrenal, possesses 1/50 of this ACTH suppression activity, while androgens and estrogens lack this ability.

Although secretion and release of aldosterone by the adrenal cortex are regulated mainly by the renin-angiotensin system and, secondarily, by plasma sodium and potassium concentrations, the availability of its biosynthetic precursors is under control of ACTH.

Renin-Angiotensin Mechanism

Renin is secreted by the juxtaglomerular cells situated next to the macula densa located at the first segment of the distal convoluted tubule. These highly specialized juxtaglomerular cells line the terminal part of the afferent arteriole just proximal to the glomerulus. The juxtaglomerular cells and the macula densa constitute the juxtagomerular apparatus. Increase in stretch of the renal arteriolar wall results in an increase in granulation in the juxta-glomerular cells, and decreased stretch is followed by degranulation of the cells and release of renin. The renal afferent arteriole functions as a stretch receptor which signals release of renin. The macula densa may serve as a volume sensor or as a chemoreceptor responsive to sodium concentration. Reduction of intravascular volume, induced by low sodium intake, blood loss, or change from recumbent to upright posture, induces a degranulation in the juxtaglomerular cells and the release of renin, a proteolytic enzyme, into the blood stream and lymph. In the blood stream, renin catalyzes the transforma-tion of a circulating globulin angiotensinogen (produced in the liver) to angiotensin I. This decapeptide is acted on by plasma angiotensin-converting enzyme with the cleavage of two amino acid residues leaving an octapeptide angiotensin II.

Angiotensin II, the most potent vasopressor agent known, also functions as the main physiologic stimulant for aldosterone release. Angiotensin II is destroyed by angiotensinases in the plasma; these enzymes may be produced in the adrenal gland. The longevity of angiotensin II in the blood stream is estimated to be 4–20 min. In addition to causing a release of aldosterone,

angiotensin II may also stimulate the release of corticosterone, desoxycorticosterone, and, to a small extent, cortisol. There are data which indicate a
mutual dependence of release of catecholamines and angiotensin II on each
other. A sufficiently low perfusion pressure in the renal arteriole induces
aldosterone release and sodium retention. Increased water reabsorption associated with this process enhances the perfusion pressure in the region of the
afferent arteriole. Macula densa chemoreceptors signal renin release when
tubular luminal sodium concentrate is low, resulting in the eventual release of
aldosterone designed to ultimately correct the hyponatremia. Reduction in
intravascular volume may induce a decrease in the inactivation of aldosterone
in the liver, resulting in increased circulating levels of aldosterone. The
synthesis of aldosterone is ultimately dependent on the presence of appropriate steroid precursors whose synthesis is ACTH-dependent. Therefore, certain
aspects of aldosterone kinetics are undoubtedly responsive to anterior pituitary function.

BIOSYNTHESIS OF ADRENOCORTICAL HORMONES

All physical signs and symptoms of adrenal disorders are reflections of
increased or decreased levels of certain biologically active hormones. The bulk
of the abnormal metabolites is biologically inactive. Discernible effects in
adrenal diseases are due to either increased or decreased glucocorticoids,
mineralocorticoids, androgens, estrogens, or combinations thereof.

The immediate precursor for corticosteriodogenesis is cholesterol. This
substrate is provided from dietary intake, as well as from synthesis from
acetyl CoA. The synthetic reaction involves the participation of several
cofactors, including pantothenic acid (for coenzyme A), NADH, and NADPH,
as well as energy from high energy phosphate bonds. The availability of
cholesterol for corticosteroidogenesis is enhanced by ACTH. At low levels of
ACTH activity, plasma cholesterol enters the synthetic pool; this action is
mediated by adenosine $3',5'$-monophosphate (cAMP) which is released from
ATP by an ACTH-activated membrane adenyl cyclase. Higher levels of ACTH
through the cAMP mechanism make cholesterol from liposomes available for
corticosteroidogenesis (Davis and Garren, 1966).

The first reaction in the corticosteroid synthetic chain is the desmolase
reaction, a multistep process which results in the cleavage of the cholesterol
side chain releasing Δ^5-pregnenolone and isocaproic acid. Pregnenolone has
two alternative fates in the biosynthetic sequence (fig. 10.1). The Δ^5, 3β-ol
structure of pregnenolone is converted to the Δ^4, 3-ketone group by a two
step microsomal reaction described as the Δ^5, 3β-ol dehydrogenase system,
resulting in the formation of progesterone. The alternative fate of pregnenolone is the hydroxylation at C 17 by a cytoplasmic 17α-hydroxylase to form

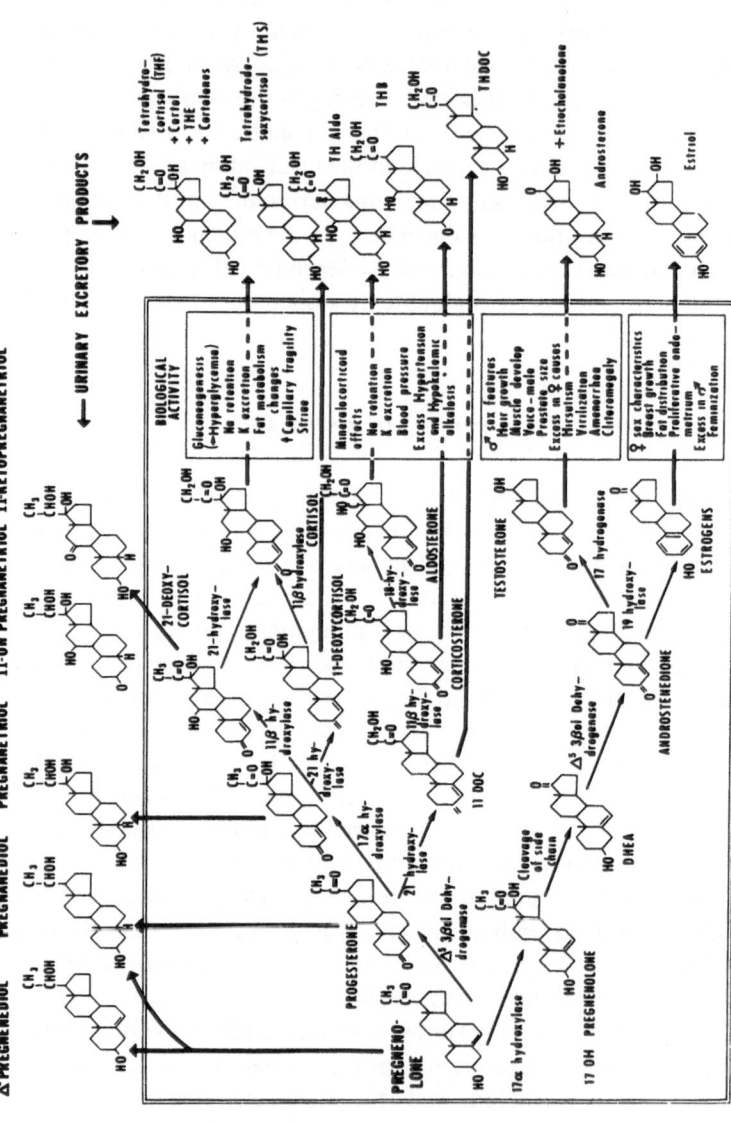

Figure 10.1. Adrenal steroidogenesis. The compound Δ⁵ pregnenolone, which is the substrate for all steroid hormone synthesis, is derived from cholesterol. ACTH activates the "desmolase" reaction which results in the formation of pregnenolone and isocaproic aldehyde. The small rectangular areas list the clinical effects of the various hormones. The compounds outside the double-lined borders are urinary end-products of the various adrenocortical steroids. Chemical properties of the end-products which are employed for quantitation are also presented. (Reprinted with permission: Bacchus, 1972.)

17α-hydroxypregnenolone. The major purpose of this pathway is synthesis of androgens and estrogens. To this end, the side chain is cleaved off, leaving a ketone group at C 17, *i.e.*, formation of Δ^5 androsten, 3β-ol, 17-one, or dehydroepiandrosterone (DHEA). As shown in figure 10.1, a microsomal Δ^5, 3β-ol dehydrogenase then converts DHEA to Δ^4 androsten, 3, 17-dione. Reduction of the 17-ketone group of androstenedione results in the formation of testosterone. Hydroxylation of androstenedione at C 19 permits subsequent aromatization of ring A of the steroid nucleus with the resulting formation of estrone, an estogen. An alternative fate of 17-hydroxypregnenolone is 17-hydroxyprogesterone as shown in figure 10.1. This 17-OH progesterone is an intermediate in the formation of cortisol. Progesterone formed from pregnenolone is the precursor to all biologically active C 21 adrenal cortical hormones. The Δ^4, 3-ketone structure is essential to the biologic activity of these hormones. Progesterone has two alternative fates in the adrenal, viz., it can be converted to 17-hydroxyprogesterone by a 17α-hydroxylase in the cytosol, or it can be converted to 11-desoxycorticosterone by a soluble 21-hydroxylase enzyme. The intermediate 17α-OH progesterone is converted to the biologically inactive intermediate 11-deoxycortisol (S) by 21-hydroxylase. A mitochondrial 11β-hydroxylase converts 11-deoxycortisol to cortisol, the definitive glucocorticoid in the human adrenal. The intermediate 11-desoxycorticosterone is converted to corticosterone by 11β-hydroxylase. The normal human adrenal produces cortisol and corticosterone in a ratio between 10:1–4:1. Corticosterone is converted to aldosterone by the enzyme 18-hydroxylase; this transformation confers powerful mineralocorticoid activity to the hormone. It is probable that, in some situations, 11β-hydroxylation may precede 21-hydroxylation (fig. 10.1).

The normal secretory rate of cortisol in the adult male is estimated to be from 20–30 mg/24 hr, and of corticosterone, from 4–6 mg/24 hr. Aldosterone secretion rate on a normal 5–10 g sodium chloride intake ranges from 60–170 μg/24 hr.

TRANSPORT OF ADRENOCORTICAL HORMONES

From 60–70% of cortisol is secreted during the period from midnight to 8:00 A.M., and the remaining 30–40% during the rest of the day. This circadian variation in cortisol secretion, evident when plasma cortisol determinations are done at 8:00 A.M. and 5:00 P.M., is obliterated in certain disease states. There is also a semblance of circadian variation of corticosterone secretion. Under maximal stimulation, the circadian variation is obliterated and the adrenal cortex can produce up to 300 mg of cortisol/24 hr.

Cortisol is transported in the circulation, bound to an α-globulin, cortisol-binding-globulin (CBG). Specific chemical characteristics in the steroid molecule are determinants of its affinity to CBG. Approximately 50–60% of cortisol is bound to CBG; and 10% circulates as free cortisol. The remainder of secreted cortisol is rapidly inactivated by the liver. The protein binding renders the hormone soluble in plasma and prevents its inactivation by the liver. Certain clinical states are associated with changes in CBG, thereby affecting cortisol kinetics. Plasma cortisol levels in the adult male range from 5–25 μg/100 ml at 8:00 A.M., and 2.5–12.5 μg/100 ml at 5:00–6:00 P.M. Plasma corticosterone levels are normally in the range of 0.5–2.5 mg/100 ml. Mean plasma concentration of aldosterone in the adult is reported to be 0.008 mg/100 ml.

FURTHER CONSIDERATIONS ON SYNTHESIS OF ANDROGENS BY THE ADRENAL CORTEX

As presented in figure 10.1 the precursor to the series is 17α-OH pregnenolone, which becomes DHEA after cleavage by a desmolase of the side chain. This compound functions as a very weak androgen, and is also a substrate for formation of androstenedione which may be hydroxylated to 11β-OH androstenedione. DHEA may be hydroxylated to C 11 to form Δ^5, androstenediol. In the adrenal cells, there is a sulfokinase which transfers sulfate to the OH group at carbon 3, hence, the formation of DHEA sulfate. A similar conjugation of testosterone, DOC, and corticosterone is possible. Cortisol, cortisone, and aldosterone are not sulfated to any significant degree.

STEROID HORMONE PRODUCTION IN FETAL ADRENALS

The fetal adrenal responds to fetal ACTH as maternal ACTH fails to traverse the placental barrier. For this reason, in an anencephalic fetus with atrophic pituitary, adrenal development does not progress beyond the twentieth week of gestation. From tenth week of gestation on, the cells destined to become the mature normal adrenals possess all the enzymes necessary for synthesis of cortisol, as well as of 17-ketosteroids. In the fetal zone of the gland, there is a deficiency in Δ^5, 3β-ol dehydrogenase system, and this could be the basis of preponderance of C 19 compounds produced by the fetus, as this fetal zone is predominant at this stage of development. Recent data reveal a unique relationship between placental HCG (chorionic gonadotropin) and the fetal zone. It is suggested that stimulation of this zone is a major function of HCG from the placenta.

BIOLOGIC ACTIONS OF ADRENOCORTICAL HORMONES

These activities will be discussed under the categories of their potencies as follows: glucocorticoids; mineralocorticoids; and androgens. The secretory rate of adrenal estrogens is small under normal conditions and does not warrant a discussion of biologic actions. For certain pathologic states, estrogen levels may be significant.

Glucocorticoids

The definitive glucocorticoid in man is cortisol, although measurable amounts of a weaker glucocorticoid, corticosterone, are also produced; corticosterone also possesses mineralocortical activity. The prime effect of cortisol is on the process of gluconeogenesis. Cortisol increases the synthesis of the enzymes essential to gluconeogenesis, *e.g.,* phosphoenol pyruvate carboxykinase (PEPCK) among others. Because of the gluconeogenic and anti-insulin actions of glucocorticoids, hyperglycemia and a metacorticoid diabetes may be induced, but this diabetic state is not usually accompanied by ketoacidosis.

Glucocorticoids also affect fat metabolism, excessive cortisol activity causing centripetal redistribution of fat. Cortisol also induces fat synthesis, partly as a result of the induced hyperglycemia which then stimulates insulin release and, eventually, lipogenesis. Chronic cortisol excess may lead to hyperlipidemia and hypercholesterolemia. Many deamination and transamination enzymes are activated by glucocorticoids.

Glucocorticoids enhance water diuresis so that, in adrenocortical insufficiency, a water load is not readily excreted. Cortisol prevents the shift of water intracellularly, hence maintaining a higher extracellular water volume. This causes a higher glomerular filtration rate and water diuresis. It has been suggested that cortisol has a direct antagonistic effect on ADH action on the renal tubule, increases ADH inactivation by the liver, and suppresses the production of ADH by the neurophypophysial system.

Glucocorticoids produce a lymphopenia by lysis of circulating and fixed lymphocytes. In this process, antibody proteins are released initially, but the continued production of antibodies is depressed by the continued thymicolymphocytolysis. Cortisol, cortisone, and aldosterone induce a depression of circulating eosinophils (and basophils) by sequestration of these cells in the lungs and spleen, and by lysis to some extent. Total neutrophils are increased by glucocorticoids, resulting in leukocytosis with neutrophilia. Glucocorticoids also stimulate erythropoiesis resulting in a pattern of steroid-induced, or stress-induced, erythrocytosis. Occasionally, cortisol-induced thrombocytosis may precipitate thromboembolic phenomena. Cortisone increases muscle performance to the extent that much activity was used in the past as an assay for glucocorticoid activity.

Glucocorticoids lower the threshold for excitation of the central nervous system; this is the basis of certain psychiatric disorders precipitated by pharmacologic doses of cortisol and similar steroids. Many patients with Cushing's syndrome exhibit psychiatric abnormalities. Pharmacologic doses of glucocorticoids result in an increase of gastric acidity, a probable decrease in protective mucopolysaccharides, and an increase in uropepsin excretion. These factors may underlie in high occurrence of peptic ulcer disease in patients treated with cortisol, or in patients under stress.

Glucocorticoids affect bone turnover by decreasing osteoblast activity and bone matrix formation (antiprotein-anabolic action), by decreasing calcium deposition, by decreasing the hepatic conversion of vitamin D to a more active biologic form, and by increasing the clearance and urinary loss of calcium. These effects of cortisol are demonstrated by the severe osteoporosis following long-term use of pharmacologic doses of cortisol, or in patients with endogenous cortisol excess such as in Cushing's syndrome.

Glucocorticoids exert effects on the cardiovascular system through different mechanisms which include an effect on sodium retention, a mineralocorticoid effect of large amounts of cortisol. Cortisol is laso known to enhance the production of angiotensinogen which would eventually lead to increased levels of angiotensin. A well-known effect of cortisol is to sensitize the vasculature to the pressor effects of catecholamines. Perhaps this sensitization action is the basis of the occasional benefits of glucocorticoid therapy in patients with shock. It is well known that decompensated cardiovascular disease is the major cause of death in Cushing's syndrome.

Glucocorticoids have been shown to possess marked anti-inflammatory effects, altering the response of connective tissues to injury. Fibroblast activity is decreased by these hormones, but fibroblast activity and the inflammatory response are increased by desoxycorticosterone, a mineralocorticoid. It is suggested that the ability of cortisol to stabilize lysosomal membranes underlies the anti-inflammatory effects of these compounds.

Biologic Actions of Mineralocorticoid Hormones

The prototype mineralocorticoid aldosterone is secreted by the zona glomerulosa of the adrenal cortex; at least two other natural steroids possess significant mineralocorticoid activity, desoxycorticosterone and corticosterone, which are produced in the human adrenal, to a small extent normally and in excessive amounts in certain pathologic states. Desoxycorticosterone possesses approximately 1/30 of the sodium-retaining potential of aldosterone, and corticosterone even less of this activity.

The major effect of aldosterone is on the reabsorption of sodium in the distal renal tubule. This permits the intracellular sodium to increase in the tubule cell, and potassium and hydrogen ions to escape into the tubular lumen. The studies of Feldman, Fundar, and Edelman (1972) revealed that aldosterone induces DNA formation and, thereby, increases extranuclear RNA production. These RNAs direct an increased synthesis of enzymes, which increases oxidative phosphorylation from carbohydrate breakdown, thereby producing sufficient intracellular high energy phosphate bonds to supply the energy for the sodium pump. Desoxycorticosterone, a less powerful mineralocorticoid, also induces a sodium retention, but it is thought to possess a somewhat higher potassium-excreting activity. The sodium retention due to aldosterone is not associated with edema, presumably because of the ability to increase gomerular filtration pressure and, thereby, water excretion. Desoxycorticosterone does not have this ability; hence, edema is often an accompaniment of excess desoxycorticosterone action.

Aldosterone has been shown to decrease carbohydrate metabolism ascribable to the associated hypokalemia. Replenishment of potassium effectively corrects this abnormal carbohydrate tolerance. It is assumed that deficiency of K^+ ions impairs the secretion and release of insulin by the β-cells of the pancreas.

Biologic Actions of Adrenal Androgens

The androgenic substances in adrenal hormone synthesis are dehydroeipandrosterone, androstenedione, and, in minimal amounts, testosterone. All except testosterone are 17-ketosteroids. These 17-KS compounds enhance amino acid incorporation into protein synthesis, and oppose the deamination and transamination catabolic reactions of glucocorticoids. Testosterone is more powerful in this regard, but the amounts produced normally in the adrenals are minimal. The effect of these adrenal 17-KS and testosterone is more important in females as they lack any other major source of androgen production. Excessive amounts of these androgens induce hirsutism, a male habitus, and clitoromegaly in females. If there is an excess of these compounds in the female fetus prior to birth, development of a male urogenital tract occurs.

CATABOLISM OF ADRENOCORTICAL SECRETIONS

As described previously, cortisol, the definitive glucocorticoid, circulates largely in a form bound to CBG, with small amounts in free form. In the presence of large amounts of cortisol production, a small fraction may be loosely bound to albumin. Conditions which alter the levels of CBG may alter the ratio of bound cortisol to free cortisol, as in patients receiving estrogens and birth control pills. Progesterone also has a strong affinity for CBG, so that, in pregnancy and in the progesterone phase of the menstrual cycle, there is sufficient displacement of cortisol from CBG to result in somewhat higher levels of free cortisol. However, during later stages of pregnancy the estrogen-induced CBG levels may be so high that the circulating total cortisol levels are elevated. In the presence of hepatocellular disease, nephrosis, amyloid disease, multiple myeloma, and congenital CBG deficiency, the levels of CBG may be low. The protein binding permits the solubility of the steroids as well as protects the steroids from inactivation by the liver. Free cortisol is readily metabolized by the liver by enzymatic reactions which render the steroid biologically inactive. The biologic half-life of cortisol is estimated to be 90 min and is prolonged in liver disease and hypothyroidism and shortened in thyrotoxicosis. The major catabolism of cortisol takes place in the liver, but the extrahepatic catabolism may be considerable under certain conditions.

Steps in Cortisol Metabolism in the Liver

The steps involved in the hepatic degradation of cortisol are similar to those involving aldosterone, cortisone, and corticosterone as well as of many of the biosynthetic intermediates. For this reason, the steps in cortisol degradation will be considered as prototype for most of the other C 21 compounds from the adrenals. There are four pathways for cortisol degradation in the liver, and perhaps in extrahepatic tissues (fig. 10.2).

(1) The first pathway involves reduction of the Δ^4, 3-ketone structure in ring A by a two step reaction, first involving Δ^4 hydrogenase and requiring NADPH, whereby cortisol is converted to dihydrocortisol, a biologically inactive compound. This reductive step is impaired in hepatocellular disease. The second step is the reduction of the ketone group at C 3 by an α-hydroxy-steroid dehydrogenase in the presence of NADH or NADPH. The resultant compound is tetrahydrocortisol, which is then conjugated to glucuronic acid at the hydroxyl group at C 3. The reaction involves the participation of uridine disphosphoglucuronic acid (UDPGA) in the presence of glucuronyl transferase, with the resulting formation of a tetrahydrocortisol glucurono-side (glucuronide) (THF glucuronide). This transformation renders the compound water-soluble, thus permitting excretion by the kidneys without any significant tubular reabsorption. This pathway of cortisol reduction amounts to approximately 45–50%.

(2) In the second pathway, a small fraction of cortisol (5–10%) is degraded to 17-ketosteroid derivatives by cleavage of the side chain. The end-products include 11β-hydroxyandrosterone and 11-ketoeticocholanolone. This pathway is also decreased in the presence of hepatocellular disease.

(3) In the third pathway, there is reduction of the ketone group at C 20 to form the glycol side chain. This reaction may precede the reduction of the Δ^4, 3-ketone group in some conditions.

(4) In the fourth pathway, there is hydroxylation of the ring structure of cortisol by certain inducible hydroxylase enzymes, e.g., 6β-hydroxylation which occurs in liver disease, pregnancy (Katz, et al., 1962), following estrogen therapy, and after phenobarbital. This pathway is not a major one normally, but may assume some significance in the clinical states described

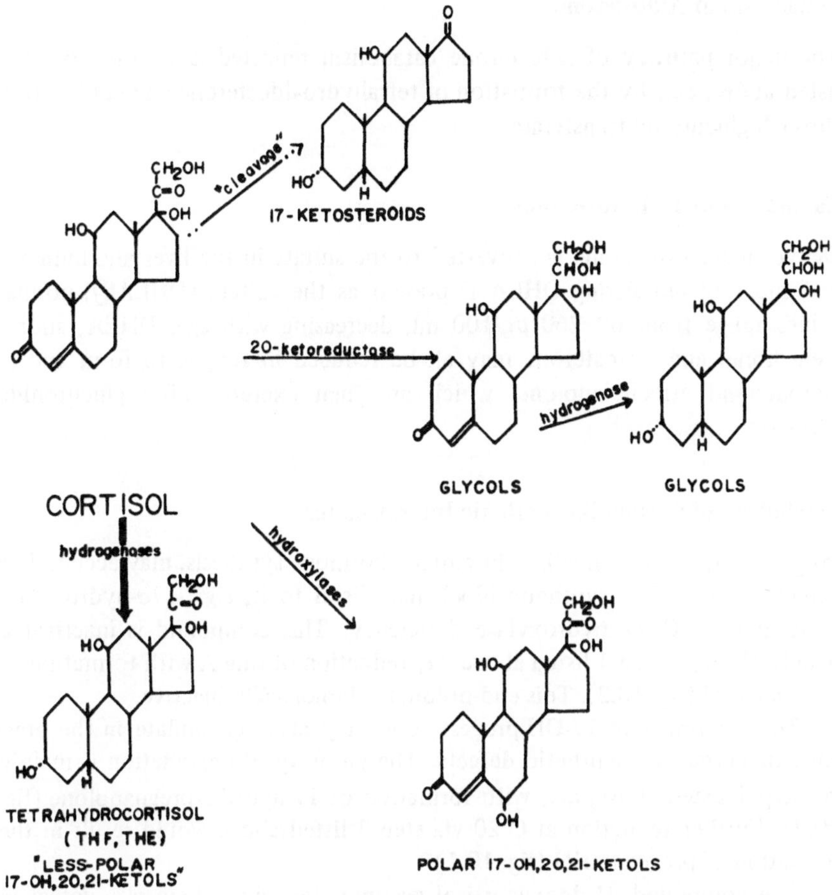

Figure 10.2. Pathways of cortisol degradation. The cleavage step involves the 17:20 desmolase reaction. Significant amounts of cortisol (F) are converted to cortisone (E). The reduction of these 11-oxygenated steroids involves a two step reaction, the end-products being THF and THE respectively. The glycol derivatives may be formed directly from cortisol without prior reduction of ring A, as well as after ring A reduction. The process of 6-hydroxylation may represent an alternative excretory pathway when THF-THE and 17-KS pathways are decreased, e.g., in hepatic cirrhosis, pregnancy, and the newborn. Enzymes involved are indicated in the figure and quantitative data are presented in the text. (Reprinted with permission: Bacchus, 1969.)

above. Under such conditions also, other hydroxylations have been known to occur. For example, the newborn infant who has significant 6β-hydroxylation pathway may also produce 2α-hydroxyl derivatives of cortisol (Ulstrom, 1960). These products are relatively water-soluble, and are excreted without prior glucuronosidation.

Catabolism of Aldosterone

The major pathway of aldosterone catabolism reported is via the first step listed above, *i.e.*, by the formation of tetrahydroaldosterone and conjugation through glucuronyl transferase.

Catabolism of 17-Ketosteroids

Dehydroepiandrosterone is converted to the sulfate in the liver and kidneys, and most of circulating DHEA is present as the sulfate (DHEAS); normal values range from 60–260 μg/100 ml, decreasing with age. DHEA, androstenedione, and testosterone may all be reduced in ring A to form androsterone and etiocholanolone, which are then excreted after glucuronide formation.

Catabolism of Certain Biosynthetic Intermediates

Progesterone, an intermediate in adrenal hormone synthesis, may accumulate whenever there is a synthetic block just distal to it, *e.g.*, 17α-hydroxylase deficiency or C 21 hydroxylase deficiency. This compound is inactivated mainly through step 1 listed above, *i.e,* reduction of ring A with formation of pregnanediol (fig. 10.2). This end-product is biologically inactive.

The intermediate 17-OH-progesterone may also accumulate in the presence of certain biosynthetic defects. The pathway of degradation is mainly via step 1 listed above, *i.e.*, with formation of 17-hydroxypregnanolone (fig. 10.2). Further reduction at C 20 via step 3 listed above would result in the formation of pregnanetriol (fig. 10.1).

The compound 21-deoxycortisol accumulates when there is a defect in 21-hydroxylation. The reduction end-product via step 1 above is 5β-pregnane-3α, 11β,17α, triol, 20-one. This, on further reduction at C 20, will result in the formation pregnane 3α,11β, 17α, 20 tetrol. It is well to note that the liver may dehydrogenate the 11-hydroxy group, with the resultant formation of 11-ketopregnanetrio (fig. 10.1).

The compound 11-deoxycortisol accumulates when there is a defect in 11β-hydroxylase, spontaneous, or induced by metyrapone. The degradation product, via step 1 above, is tetrahydrocortisol (THS) (fig. 10.3), which is excreted as the glucuronide. In the presence of very large amounts of this compound, additional step 1 results in the formation of pregnan 3, 17, 20, 21 tetrol.

The compound corticosterone (B) may occur in the presence of 17α-hydroxylase deficiency in man. The degradation pathway is mainly via step 1 above, to tetrahydrocorticosterone (THB), which is then excreted as the glucuronide or sulfate.

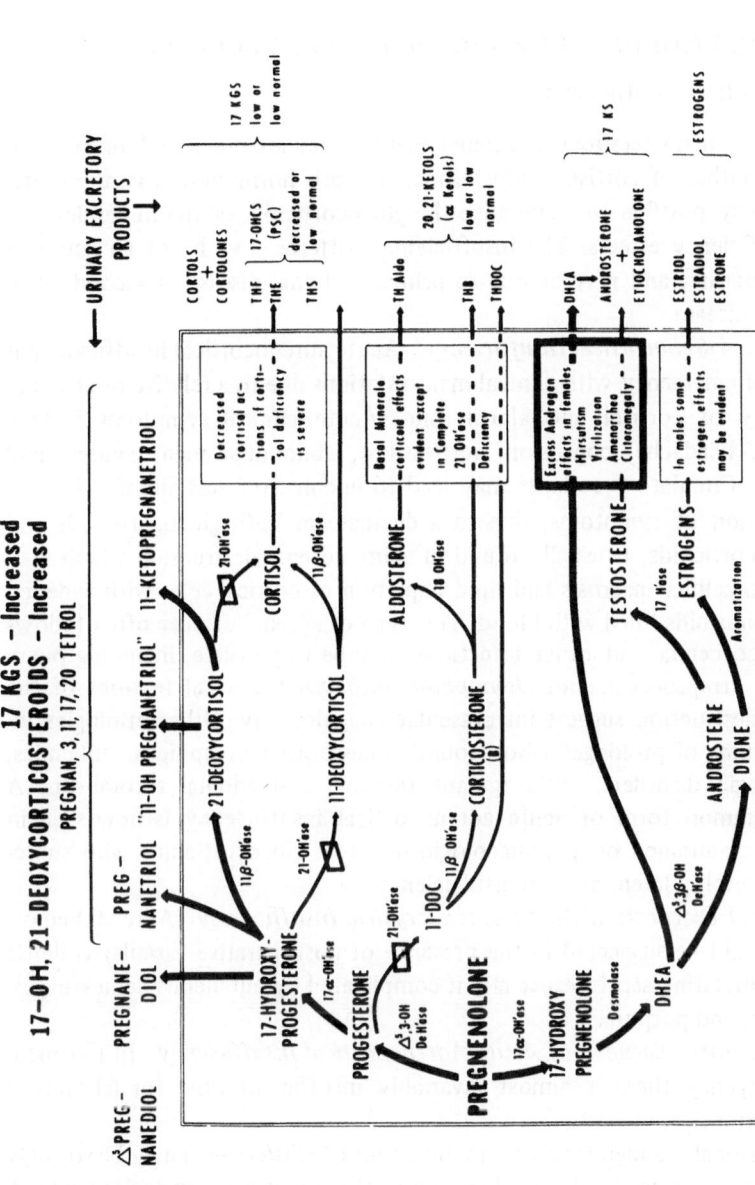

Figure 10.3. Clinical features and pattern of corticosteroid metabolites found in adrenocortical 21-hydroxylase deficiency. Pregnanetriol and 11-ketopregnanetriol, among others, are increased in this defect. Clinical manifestations are listed in the rectangular boxes. Urinary end-products are depicted outside the double-lined rectangle, and chemical procedures for their detection are listed. (Reprinted with permission: Bacchus, 1972).

Desoxycorticosterone (DOC), similar to corticosterone, is excreted as tetrahydrodesoxycorticosterone (THDOC) glucuronide or as the sulfate.

CLINICAL DISORDERS OF ADRENOCORTICAL FUNCTION

Adrenocortical Insufficiency

The clinical manifestations of adrenal insufficiency are due to a deficiency, or absence, either of cortisol, aldosterone, or both hormones. It is, therefore, occasionally possible to distinguish the glucocorticoid, or the mineralocorticoid, deficiency effects. The insufficiency patterns may be of an acute or chronic nature, and may be due to primary adrenal disease or secondary to pituitary disease.

Acute Adrenocortical Insufficiency Acute adrenocortical insufficiency is a medical emergency with clinical manifestations due to a relative or absolute deficiency of cortisol and aldosterone. Acute clinical symptoms include lassitude, headache, confusion, restlessness, abdominal pain, nausea, and vomiting. Circulatory collapse may lead to unconsciousness and shock. This constellation of symptoms, due to a decrease in both glucocorticoids and mineralocorticoids, is usually found in acute adrenal destruction which may be due to cellular necrosis and lipid depletion of cortical cells, with widened adrenal sinusoids filled with blood. This type of adrenal damage often follows meningococcemia, but other infections may be responsible, including pneumococci, streptococci, and *Hemophilus influenzae*. Several features of the adrenal destruction suggest intravascular coagulopathy. Other etiologies include trauma of prolonged labor (found in newborns), pemphigus, leukemias, hemorrhagic disorders, anticoagulant therapy, and adrenal thrombosis. A fairly common form of acute adrenocortical insufficiency is now seen in patients maintained on pharmacologic doses of glucocorticoids who subsequently develop latent adrenal insufficiency.

Clinical Diagnosis of Acute Adrenocortical Insufficiency Adrenal hemorrhage should be suspected in the presence of postoperative vascular collapse or of fulminating sepsis, especially if complicated by cutaneous hemorrhages, petechiae, and purpura.

Laboratory Diagnosis of Acute Adrenocortical Insufficiency In this medical emergency there is almost invariably insufficient time for laboratory confirmation.

Occasionally a high total eosinophil count (> 50/cu mm) may be strongly suggestive, since, in shock of other causes, there is usually an eosinopenia. A serum sodium:potassium ratio is occasionally helpful if it drops from the usual 30 toward 20. It is occasionally possible to measure serum cortisol by the fluorimetric method, as an emergency procedure. In adrenocortical insufficiency, the values are low or normal, whereas, in shock of another cause, the adrenals are capable of increasing cortisol release by several-fold. It is suggested that suspected cases be treated with glucocorticoids after a plasma sample is obtained for cortisol determination which is to be done later.

Chronic Adrenocortical Insufficiency Chronic adrenocortical insufficiency may be due to primary adrenal disease, or secondary to pituitary insufficiency. The spectrum of disorders includes general adrenocortical failure, isolated hypoaldosteronism, or isolated decrease in cortisol and 17-KS, such as in adrenal insufficiency following exogenous steroid therapy.

Addison's Disease (Primary Chronic Adrenocortical Insufficiency) Cited in Forsham (1969), Addison's disease directed attention to "anemia, general languor and debility, remarkable feebleness of the heart's action, irritability of the stomach, and a peculiar change in the color of the skin." All manifestations in that description, except for the pigmentary changes, are due to deficiency in the cortical hormones which is also the basis of weakness and fatiguability, weight loss and dehydration, hypotension, small heart, anorexia, nausea, vomiting, diarrhea and epigastric pain, dizziness, syncopal attacks, nervousness, mental changes, and occasionally, hypoglycemic symptoms. Some patients may complain of muscle cramps and salt-craving, and may have flexion contractures of the hands. Etiologies of Addison's disease include: (1) idiopathic atrophy of the adrenals, possibly on an autoimmune basis (50–60% of cases are in this group); (2) tuberculosis (accounting for 30–40% of cases); and rarer causes, such as histoplasmosis, metastatic disease, hemochromatosis, amyloidosis, and vascular accidents. Many patients with autoimmune adrenocortical insufficiency have been observed to have amenorrhea, presumably due to an autoimmune disorder against other steroid-producing cells. Associated disorders include Schmidt's syndrome (adrenal insufficiency, thyroiditis, and diabetes), as well as hypoparathyroidism with adrenal insufficiency and cutaneous moniliasis.

Laboratory Diagnosis of Chronic Adrenocortical Insufficiency The availability of sensitive methods for measurement of plasma cortisol and urinary corticosteroids makes it unnecessary to depend on indirect tests, but two indirect tests, because of their relative reliability and simplicity, are recommended in screening for adrenal insufficiency. These tests are the water diuresis test, in which a failure to excrete over 1,000 ml of ingested 1,500 ml of water is considered as compatible with adrenal insufficiency, and the serum sodium:potassium ratio is lower than 30 and approaches 20 in adrenal insufficiency, probably a reflection of mineralocorticoid deficiency. The direct procedures include study of plasma cortisol and responsiveness to corticotropin stimulation, and urinary steroids and the responsiveness to similar stimulation. The following sequence of studies is recommended. The first procedure is plasma cortisol response to intravenous cosyntropin. An adequate increment in plasma cortisol after cosyntropin effectively rules out adrenocortical insufficiency. The absence of significant increase in plasma cortisol is compatible with adrenocortical insufficiency. In this case, it is useful to repeat the test with repeat injections at 1-hr intervals for 3 doses, at which intervals there should be progressive increases in plasma cortisol in patients with latent adrenal insufficiency. Failure to obtain incremental increases would be compatible with primary adrenal insufficiency. The second procedure, the repeated 8-hr intravenous ACTH test, is a more cumbersome alternative procedure, in which failure of significant incremental increases in urinary 17-OHCS in 17-KGS would be compatible with primary adrenal insufficiency. Incremental increases after repeated challenges would suggest secondary adrenal insufficiency.

Secondary Adrenocortical Insufficiency Secondary adrenocortical insufficiency may occur as part of a multiglandular deficiency of ACTH. The clinical manifestations in adrenocortical insufficiency secondary to panhypopituitarism are similar to Addison's disease, except for the lack of pigmentation, but will be complicated by evidence of other hormonal deficiencies, *e.g.*, an associated hypometabolism, coarse skin, alopecia and bradycardia with hypothyroidism; and decreased libido, decrease in pubic and axillary hair, amenorrhea, and atrophic vaginal changes in the female with hypogonadism. Isolated ACTH deficiency is similar to Addison's disease, except for an absence of pigmentation and a less marked defect in mineral metabolism.

In the laboratory workup for this type of clinical problem, the following studies are recommended. The vasopressin stimulation test is a relatively simple procedure based on the ability of vasopressin either to act as a corticotropin-releasing factor, or to stimulate release of CRF. Increases in plasma cortisol after vasopressin challenge would effectively rule out pituitary ACTH insufficiency. A failure to increase plasma cortisol, in the face of good response to intravenous cosyntropin, would be compatible with pituitary ACTH deficiency. The metyrapone test, by either intravenous infusion (30 mg/kg in 500 ml of normal saline over a 4-hr period) or ingestion of tablets (750 mg every 4 hr for 24 hr) monitored by urinary 17-OHCS, 17-KGS, or 11-deoxy, -17-OHCS, is another recommended study. A more rapid procedure is to give the patient 750 mg of metyrapone with an antacid, orally at midnight, and check that the plasma level of 11-deoxycortisol greater than 4 ng/100 ml is compatible with normal pituitary adrenal axis function (Forsham, 1969). Pituitary ACTH deficiency should be considered in a patient who exhibits significant adrenal response to repeat ACTH (or cosyntropin) challenges and fails to exhibit a significant increase in the steroid parameters after metyrapone administration. The third procedure, plasma cortisol response to insulin hypoglycemia, is essentially similar to that for GH response (Chapter 3), except that cortisol levels are monitored in this procedure. (In most cases, it is recommended that both plasma GH and cortisol should be measured during this test, as it is often necessary to determine multiple pituitary functions.) A normal response is a doubling of the plasma cortisol, or an increment of at least 7 μg/100 ml when baseline cortisol is low. Lack of such response, in a patient who responded adequately to cosyntropin, would be consistent with pituitary ACTH deficiency or with lack of hypothalamic CRF response.

Treatment of Adrenocortical Insufficiency

Acute Adrenocortical Insufficiency The immediate goals in the treatment of acute adrenal insufficiency are to replace fluids to combat dehydration and shock, replace cortisol, and identify the precipitating cause. Vital signs should be monitored continuously or at least every 30 min.

An infusion of 5% glucose in normal saline is started. Additional solutions may be infused through the tubing.

Soluble cortisol (as hemisuccinate) is given intravenously at the dose range of 100–200 mg (in adults) immediately, to be followed by 50–100 mg every 2–4 hr thereafter. Such high doses at these intervals are necessary because of the short biologic half-life of this water-soluble cortisol preparation. If there is continued shock, the potent pressor agent, angiotensin II (available as Hypertensin-Schering), should be employed in preference to norepinephrine or metaraminol. If the precipitating cause is identified, appropriate treatment should be instituted at this time.

On the second day, if the patient has stabilized to some degree, cortisone acetate may be substituted by mouth at the dosage of 50 mg/day if oral intake is possible. Otherwise, cortisol hemisuccinate (100–150 mg/day) may be given parenterally. With further stabilization, the patient may be continued on a regular diet with adequate sodium chloride, and given between 25–37.5 mg of cortisone acetate orally daily as the maintenance dose in chronic adrenocorticol insufficiency. It is recommended that the minerolocorticoid 9α-fluorocortisol be given orally, at the dose range of 0.1 mg daily. The correct dosage may be monitored by serum or urine potassium values.

Treatment of Chronic Adrenocortical Insufficiency The therapeutic goals are maintenance of blood volume and restoration of strength, weight, blood pressure, hemoglobin, and blood sugar to essentially normal levels. Cortisol or cortisone acetate are given in replacement dosages (25 mg–37.5 mg daily). Patients who have laboratory or clinical evidence of mineralocorticoid insufficiency are given 0.05 mg–0.2 mg of 9α-fluorocortisol daily, the adequacy of the dosage being monitored by serum or urine electrolytes. Excessive dosages of this mineralocorticoid may result in edema, headaches, hypertension, contractures of tendons, and hypokalemia. Because of the nature of this chronic disorder, the patient should carry a "dog-tag" indicating the diagnosis. Intercurrent stresses or infections may require increased steroid dosages.

Treatment of Secondary Adrenocortical Insufficiency The management of the adrenocortical insufficiency component of this disorder requires replacement doses of cortisol or cortisone acetate. Mineralocorticoid replacement is required very rarely. The other target gland deficiencies should be treatment with replacement doses of thyroxin or triiodothyronine (for thyroid), testosterone propionate or cypionate (for male gonadal insufficiency), and estrogens (for female gonadal insufficiency).

Diseases of Adrenocortical Hyperfunction

Hypercortisol and hyperaldosterone disorders will be discussed in this section. Biosynthetic defects in the adrenals will be discussed in a separate section.

Cushing's Syndrome   Cushing's syndrome is a relatively rare disorder, but there are series which suggest a prevalence of 1 in every 1,000 autopsies. It is described as three to four times more common in women than in men. The peak incidence is described at between 20–40 yr, but the disease has been found in younger as well as older patients. The syndrome is due to excess adrenal hormones, mainly cortisol, whether due to nonpathologic states such as chronic stress or to three groups of pathologic processes, viz., excessive pituitary ACTH with adrenocortical hyperplasia, autonomous adrenocortical neoplasia, or ectopic production of ACTH with consequent adrenal hyperplasia. The adrenals of approximately 10% of patients with Cushing's syndrome show no overt pathology, 60% show hypertrophy and hyperplasia, and 30% show tumors, of which one-half are benign and somewhat less than half are malignant. A relatively rare cause is nodular hyperplasia which may be autonomous.

In Cushing's syndrome due to excess ACTH, most of the patients have a defect in the regulation of the hypothalamus-pituitary-axis as the hypothalamic corticotropin-releasing factor mechanism is not responsive to feedback inhibition by circulating cortisol. About 10% of this group have ACTH-secreting tumors, either small basophilic adenomas or larger chromophobe adenomas. Patients with bilateral adrenal hyperplasia, who were treated by bilateral adrenalectomy, may develop chromophobe or basophilic adenomas, some appearing years after the adrenalectomy. These patients secrete large amounts of ACTH, and may show considerable amounts of pigmentation. In the patients with adrenocortical hyperplasia, the zona glomerulosa is usually spared of marked histologic changes.

In Cushing's syndrome due to adrenocortical neoplasia, approximately 30% of the patients have autonomous adrenal tumors, in most cases, benign adenomas, and, less frequently, carcinomas. The cortisol produced by these tumors suppresses ACTH activity, and as a consequence, the contralateral adrenal as well as nontumorous adrenal tissue contiguous with the tumor become atrophic. Over 100 cases of Cushing's syndrome due to ectopic ACTH production have been reported associated with a variety of nonadrenal malignant neoplasms. This disorder has been most frequently reported in association with anaplastic small cell bronchogenic carcinoma, but it has also been seen in association with pancreatic tumors, malignant thymomas, thyroid and ovarian carcinoma, bronchial adenoma, as well as with other malignant neoplasms.

The major manifestations of Cushing's syndrome are due to hypercortisolemia. These include changes in carbohydrate, protein, and fat metabolism, leading to muscle wasting, centripetal redistribution of body fat with cervicodorsal fat pad, moon facies, and pendulous abdomen. The skin is thin, with atrophic subutaneous tissues, and, superimposed, on this is an erythrocytosis, hence, the plethoric appearance. Purple striae in the abdomen, back, and breasts also appear. Increased capillary fragility is the basis of easy bruisability and abrasions. The hypercortisolemia is also the basis of decreased osteoblastic activity and decreased bone matrix, with resulting osteoporosis. This may give rise to back pain and deformities in the spine. Demineralization of the skull is also a feature in the syndrome.

Approximately 90% of these patients exhibit glucose intolerance, but they are not prone to ketoacidosis. An increase in arteriosclerosis in these patients has been ascribed to hyperlipidemia, but hypertension may also be a factor. Hirsutism and acne are due to an increased production of androgens by the hyperplasic adrenals. Approximately less than 10% of patients with Cushing's syndrome may show an elevation of aldosterone with resultant hypokalemic alkalosis.

It has been suggested by Forsham (1969) that the presence of three or more of the following symptoms strongly suggest Cushing's syndrome: extreme weakness and muscle wasting, obesity with centripetal fat distribution, marked growth arrest in children, red and linear striae, ecchymoses in the presence of normal platelet counts, hypertension, osteoporosis, and hyperglycemic glucose tolerance tests. Sudden onset of symptoms would suggest an adenoma or adrenocarcinoma; slower progression should suggest bilateral adrenal hyperplasia.

Laboratory Diagnosis of Cushing's Syndrome The typical patient with Cushing's syndrome will show a leukocytosis with relative lymphopenia, and neutrophilia and eosinopenia. Most of these patients will also have an erythrocytosis with hematocrits of 50% or greater. Either an elevated fasting or postprandial blood sugar is also suggestive, as is a diabetic type glucose tolerance curve. About 10–15% of patients with Cushing's syndrome (especially associated with ectopic ACTH or adenocarcinoma of the adrenal) have a hypokalemic alkalosis despite normal aldosterone levels.

Definitive tests in hypercortisolemia syndromes include: (1) plasma cortisol levels (samples drawn at 8:00 A.M. and 5:00 P.M. are higher than 25 μg/100 ml and reveal lack of normal circadian variation); and (2) one dose overnight dexamethasone suppression test (the 8:00 A.M. plasma cortisol, after receiving 1.0 mg of dexamethasone the previous 11:00 P.M., is below 5

Table 10.1. Laboratory Differentiation of Cushing's Syndrome

Test	Normal	Hyperplasia	Adenoma	Carcinoma
17-Hydroxycorticosteroids (17-OHCS)	2.5–8mg/24 hr	↑ (14)	↑ (25–30)	↑↑ (50+)
ACTH stimulation	↑↑ (2–4x)	↑↑↑ (4x)	↑↑↑ (4x)	No increment
Dexamethasone suppression				
Light (2 mg/day for 3 days)	↓ (0.5x)	No change	No change	No change
Heavy (8 mg/day for 3 days)	↘ (0.5x)	↘ (0.5x)	No change	No change
17-Ketogenic steroids	8–18 mg/24 hr	↑ (2x)	↑ (2x)	↑↑↑ (10x)
ACTH stimulation	↑↑ (2x)	↑↑ (2–3x)	↑↑ (2–3x)	No increment
Dexamethasone suppression				
Light	↓ (0.5x)	No change	No change	No change
Heavy	→	→	No change	No change
17-Ketosteroids	7–15 mg/24 hr	↑ (20)	↑ or normal	↑↑↑ (6x)
ACTH stimulation	↑ (2x)	↑ (2x)	↑ (2x)	No increment
Dexamethasone suppression				
Light	↘	No change	No change	No change
Heavy	↘ (0.5x)	↘ (0.5x)	No change	No change

μg/100 ml in normal subjects, and < 10 μg/100 ml in obese subjects. Patients with Cushing's syndrome show plasma cortisol levels of > 10 μg/100 ml). (Additional studies in the differential diagnosis of hypercortisolemic syndromes are presented in table 10.1.)

Treatment of Cushing's Syndrome   Bilateral adrenocortical hyperplasia causing Cushing's syndrome is most effectively treated by bilateral adrenalectomy. After extirpation of the glands, replacement therapy with cortisol or cortisone acetate is imperative. Higher doses are required initially postoperatively, followed by maintenance doses of cortisol (30 mg/day) or of cortisone acetate in equivalent doses. Addition of 9α-fluorohydrocortisone (0.05 mg– 0.1 mg daily) is often required for mineralocortocoid replacement. Approximately 10% of patients treated by surgery may be found a few years later to have basophilic or chromophobe adenomas of the pituitary which may be locally invasive, affecting the visual fields. Hyperpigmentation is a frequent accompaniment in this disorder (Nelson's syndrome).

Cushing's syndrome due to adrenocortical adenoma is treated surgically, either by resections of the tumor or by unilateral adrenalectomy. Because of atrophy of the remaining nontumorous adrenal tissue, short-term ACTH stimulation is occasionally employed. The patients may need low dose cortisol replacement until the remaining adrenal tissue becomes active.

In the presence of pituitary overactivity irradiation or cryosurgery, yttrium implants may be helpful. Pituitary tumors are treated by surgical hypophysectomy. Replacement therapy of the target endocrine gland functions (if thyroid, adrenals, and gonadal) is imperative.

Medical management of Cushing's syndrome may be employed in functioning adrenocortical carcinoma. Effective agents include aminoglutethimide, o,p, D D D (1,1, dichloro-2-(O-chlorophenyl)-2-(p-chlorophenyl ethane), amphenone, and metryapone. These agents block adrenocortical hormone synthesis.

Diseases of Mineralocorticoid Excess

A small number of patients with Cushing's syndrome may exhibit manifestations of aldosterone excess, viz., hypokalemic hypochloremic alkalosis and some elevation in urinary aldosterone. In some of these patients, there is also an elevation of the nonaldosterone mineralocorticoids, corticosterone, and desoxycorticosterone, a result of hypernormal adrenocortical biosynthetic pathways.

Primary Hyperaldosteronism   In 1955, Conn described a syndrome consisting of arterial hypertension, hypokalemic alkalosis, and muscle weakness, associated with vasopressin-resistant polyuria, which he proved to be due to an excess of aldosterone produced by an adrenocortical tumor. The current estimate is that aldosterone-producing tumors, in contrast to hyperplasia, are now the most common form of adrenocortical origin. Aldosterone tumors are usually benign, solitary canary-yellow, containing cells resembling the zona glomerulosa. These tumors may also secrete increased amounts of cortico-sterone and DOC.

Major clinical manifestations of primary hyperaldosteronism include hypertension, hypokalemia, polyuria, polydipsia, alkalosis, albuminuria, paresthesias, and periodic paralysis. Edema is present only as a complication of hypertension; sodium retention in this state permits an increased glomerular filtration, and there is an escape from sodium-induced edema. Hypokalemia is often a late sign of this problem, and it may be antedated by hypertension by years (Conn, 1965). There is a relative paucity of retinal arterial disease seen in these patients. Severe headaches may be a manifestation of hypertension.

Decreased total exchangeable potassium is present in all patients with aldosteronism, despite occasional normal serum potassium values. Hypokalemia is more likely to occur when the sodium intake is normal or high, and may be normalized when the sodium intake is low. Hypokalemia is responsible for a fluctuating muscle weakness, postural hypotension, and a peculiar type of tetany (positive Trousseau's and Chvostek's signs) seen more frequently during potassium repletion. Renal concentration defects may result from hypokalemic tubular nephropathy.

Secondary Hyperaldosteronism   Excessive and occasionally inappropriate overproduction of aldosterone is observed in some edematous states such as hepatic cirrhosis, nephrosis, and congestive heart failure, occasionally during salt deprivation, in hypovolemia, and in malignant hypertension. Secondary hyperaldosteronism is regularly associated with nephrosis, cirrhosis, and almost invariably with malignant hypertension, other edematous states showing variable increases. Decreased intravascular volume in edematous states induces a release of renin which increases the production of angiotensin, with subsequent activation of the zona glomerulosa to produce increased amounts of aldosterone; subsequent hypernatremia exacerbates the edema. Increased aldosterone secretion during salt deprivation is a compensatory mechanism to aid in retaining sodium. Aldosteronemia in malignant hypertension is secondary to a rise in renin secretion. The most common etiologies in this type of hypertension are intrarenal vascular obstruction and intrarenal lesions not involving large renal occlusion. The clinical picture seen in secondary hyperaldosteronism is similar to that in the primary form complicated by the underlying cause, *e.g.,* edema and hepatic disease.

Nonaldosterone Hypermineralocorticoid Syndromes   These include the bisoynthetic defects in the adrenal cortex such as: (1) 17α-hydroxylase deficiency with increased corticosterone and DOC causing hypertension and hypokalemic alkalosis; hypogonadism is due to decreased androgen release secondary to the biosynthetic defect in the adrenal; (2) 11β-hydroxylase deficiency with hypertension and hypokalemic alkalosis due to accumulation of DOC; virilization noted in this state is due to increased androgen release secondary to the biosynthetic defect in the adrenal; and (3) accumulation of 18-hydroxycorticosterone due to a biosynthetic defect in the adrenals. These will be discussed in another section.

Laboratory Tests in the Diagnosis of Hypermineralocorticoid States   The sodium loading test (oral) and the intravenous sodium chloride tests may be monitored by the serum potassium levels; in patients with hyperaldosteronism, the high sodium intake is followed by a decrease in serum potassium to 3.5 mEq/L or lower. The spironolactone test is best done in patients with hypokalemia. The administration of spironolactone to patients with hyperaldosteronism and hypokalemia is followed by an increase in serum potassium of greater than 1 mEq/L.

Tests Involving Measurement of Urinary or Plasma Aldosterone   In the first test, plasma aldosterone is measured after sodium loading procedures (2 L of normal saline in 3 hr) and the levels are compared to levels in a baseline plasma sample. In hyperaldosteronism, the sodium loading procedure fails to induce a reduction in plasma aldosterone levels. (Urinary excretion of aldosterone may be measured in this procedure also.)

In the second test, desoxycorticosterone (DOC) suppression test, injection of 5 mg of DOC acetate 4 times daily or oral intake of 0.1 mg 9α-fluorocortisol 4 times daily is followed by a decrease in plasma aldosterone levels in normal subjects. Initially high values in primary aldosteronism are essentially unaltered.

In the third test, plasma renin activity (PRA) responses to challenges in posture and salt intake are helpful in distinguishing aldosteronism associated with high PRA (secondary) and with low PRA (primary).

The fourth test, adrenal venography and cannulation for aldosterone levels in adrenal veins, is usually employed in patients with aldosterone excess. The affected adrenal and location of the tumors may be identified. It is well to note, however, that most aldosteronomas are less than 3 cm in diameter.

Treatment of Hyperaldosteronism   Aldosterone-producing tumors are resected surgically. These patients may suffer a temporary hypoaldosteronism soon after surgery. Mild cases of normokalemic primary hyperaldosteronism with mild hypertension are treated with spironolactone. Rare cases of ACTH-dependent aldosteronism associated with adrenal hyperplasia are treated with ACTH suppressive doses of dexamethasone.

IDIOPATHIC CYCLIC EDEMA

Idiopathic cyclic edema is a syndrome characterized by cyclic or recurrent accumulation of extracellular fluid in which sodium and chloride are the principal electrolyte constituents. The major clinical manifestations include a periodic, but not necessarily regular, distension of the face, hands, and feet by a brawny nonpitting type of edema. The disorder most often affects overweight women of the middle-age, who may also complain of abdominal distension. In many patients, the edema may coincide with premenstrual tension, but the menstrual cycle is probably not etiologically related to the syndrome as it may also be found in menopausal patients. Patients with this disorder may also complain of headache anxiety, depression, and increased irritability. In severely affected patients, the weight may increase by up to 6 kg in a single day, but the usual gain is about 1–3 kg. Many patients may exhibit signs of hypokalemia, postural hypotension, and hypomagnesemia, all ascribable to excessive use of diuretics in attempts to control the edematous state. Because of the progression of the edema as the day wears on, the syndrome is often termed postural edema. The edema is considerably less severe while the patient is in a recumbent position, and it is markedly positively correlated with physical activity. The disorder is usually self-limited, and is not known to progress to any more serious disease. Some patients may intermittently suffer from the symptoms for 10–20 yr.

The etiology of this syndrome is not clear, but several aspects of its pathogenesis are known. There is convincing evidence that there is a component of increased capillary permeability with loss of fluid and albumin into the extravascular compartment. Decreased vascular volume induces an increased release of catecholamines and degranulation of the juxtaglomerular apparatus resulting in release of renin. This enzyme then converts angiotensinogen to angiotensin, which activates the secretion and release of aldosterone from the zona glomerulosa of the adrenal cortex. The aldosterone release, therefore, represents a compensatory mechanism. But is has been suggested that a component of hyperresponsiveness of the renin-angiotensin mechanism may be involved. It is not likely that the entire disorder is precipitated by hyperaldosteronism, as typically primary aldosteronism is not complicated by edema, because of participation of the hypothetical "third factor" or by compensatory hemodynamic alterations.

Several metabolic and hemodynamic studies demonstrated that the patient with idiopathic cyclic edema responds quite appropriately to changes in salt intake if the salt is given over a span of time. Sodium excretion after saline infusion was slower than in normal subjects, however. Rovner et al. (1972) concluded that patients with idiopathic cyclic edema do not adapt well to rapid changes in salt intake, and it was suggested that this may well be the major pathogenetic mechanism. The possibility of microvascular disease as the basis of this syndrome has been suggested by some studies, but this concept has not been definitively proved.

There are several pieces of evidence against the concept that idiopathic cyclic edema is a variant of the syndrome of inappropriate secretion of antidiuretic hormone (SIADH). Patients with SIADH exhibit hypo-osmolar plasma, hyperosmolar urine, low serum chloride, and sodium, none of which is found in patients with cyclic edema.

Diagnosis of this disorder is made only after other etiologies of edema are eliminated. It is, therefore, important to check the status of renal function by a creatinine clearance test, and occasionally, by biopsy. Liver and cardiac diseases should be excluded by the appropriate methods. The presence of hypoalbuminemia and hyperglobulinemia should be ruled out also. The key features of the diagnosis include the presence of brawny edema, indicating extravasation of protein, wide fluctuations in body weight within a single day, and considerably less severe symptoms while the patient is in a recumbent position. Serum sodium and chloride should be normal except if the patient had been on diuretics, in which case the serum potassium is also low. Albumin turnover studies reveal a more rapid loss of infused albumin into the extravascular compartment.

Treatment of idiopathic cyclic edema is not completely satisfactory. Some patients have found some degree of relief after the use of dextroamphetamine, which supposedly decreases vascular permeability and also alleviates the depressed state seen in some patients. Occasional combinations of dextroamphetamine and amytal have been helpful. Physical procedures, such as the use of abdominal binding and support hose, have been of help in some patients, but these methods are considered cumbersome by most. Several workers recommend the use of relatively small amounts of spironolactone to oppose the effect of the secondary aldosteronism component of the disorder. The patient should be reassured as to the eventual outlook in this syndrome.

CLINICAL SYNDROMES DUE TO BIOSYNTHETIC DEFECTS IN THE ADRENAL CORTEX

This group of clinical disorders is most simply considered in the context of the biosynthetic scheme presented in figure 10.1. The clinical manifestations are due to effects of the accumulation of compounds proximal to the biosynthetic defect; greatest accumulation occurs in the compound (or compounds) which is the immediate substrate for the blocked reaction. In view of the biosynthetic blocks in the adrenal cortex, it is expected that there should always be a decreased level of cortisol in such patients. Indeed, this occurs often, the plasma cortisol or urinary 11-oxy 17-OHCS being low or at the lower normal limits, but in most cases there is a compensatory reaction, whereby a large amount of substrate aids in inducing some enzymatic conversion. The most common forms of the biosynthetic problems involve steps late in the sequence, viz., 21-hydroxylase deficiency and 11β-hydroxylase defi-

Table 10.2. Summary of Clinical Features in Adrenocortical Biosynthetic Defects

Clinical features	20α-desmolase defect	3β-hydroxysteroid dehydrogenase defect	17α-hydroxylase defect	11β-hydroxylase defect	21α-hydroxylase defect
Hyperkalemic crises	Present	Present	Absent	Absent	Present in complete form
Hypertension	Absent	Absent	Present due to DOC	Present due to DOC	Absent
Secondary sex characteristics	Female	Female with clitoromegaly; ambiguous in male	Female in XX; ambiguous in XY	Ambiguous in XX; male in XY	Ambiguous in XX; male in XY
Postnatal virilization	Sexual infantilism at puberty	Mild due to DHEA	Sexual infantilism at puberty	Present	Present

ciency. Other deficiencies, *e.g.*, 17α-hydroxylase, Δ^5, 3β-ol dehydrogenase, and demolase, occur less frequently and are rapidly fatal unless diagnosed early. All of these defects are associated with adrenocortical hyperplasia; the hypocortisolemia induces increased ACTH release and continued stimulation of the adrenal cortex. The various disorders are detailed below and summarized in table 10.2.

Adrenocortical Hyperplasia Due to C 21 Hydroxylase Deficiency

This is the most common form of adrenocortical hyperplasia due to biosynthetic defect, and it may be congenital in origin with manifestations quite early in development or may become overt postpubertally. The defect may be partial (more frequent) or complete (*e.g.*, salt-losing form of CAH), in which insufficient amounts of aldosterone are produced. The difference between the affinity of 17α-OH progesterone and progesterone for 21-hydroxylase may well explain presence of aldosterone production in the non-salt-losing form. The scheme in figure 10.3 depicts accumulation of 17-hydroxyprogesterone and 21-deoxycortisol; 17-OH progesterone may serve as a precursor of weak 17-KS androgens, but there is also retrograde piling up and accumulation of compounds formed from alternate pathways, *e.g.*, C 19-androgens from the androgen pathway. The androgen effects depend on the age of the individual at the time critical levels are achieved; malformations around the urogenital sinus and external genitalia may occur in early onset of the defect. If the critical levels are achieved later, then the manifestations include hirsutism, clitoromegaly, and amenorrhea. Figure 10.3 also reveals that the major urinary steroids which accumulate in this defect are pregnanetriol, 11-keto-pregnanetriol, pregnanolone, and pregnan 3, 11, 17, 20 tetrol.

Adrenocortical Hyperplasia Due to 11β-Hydroxylase Deficiency

A lack of decrease of the 11β-hydroxylating enzyme results in accumulation of 11-desoxycorticosol (S) and its reduction product THS, which are biologically inactive. The defect also leads to an accumulation of 11-deoxycorticosterone, a powerful mineralocorticoid, hence the occurrence of hypertension (hypertensive congenital adrenal hyperplasia (HCAH)), and hypokalemic alkalosis. Hirsutism, pseudohermaphroditism, and macrogenitosomia also occur, the results of androgenic derivatives of the precursors and of steroids from alternate biosynthetic pathways. Pigmentation also occurs due to increased ACTH. The compounds which accumulate in this defect include THS, its 20-reduced derivative pregnan 3, 17, 20, 21 tetrol, and 17-ketosteroids from enhanced alternative pathways (fig. 10.4).

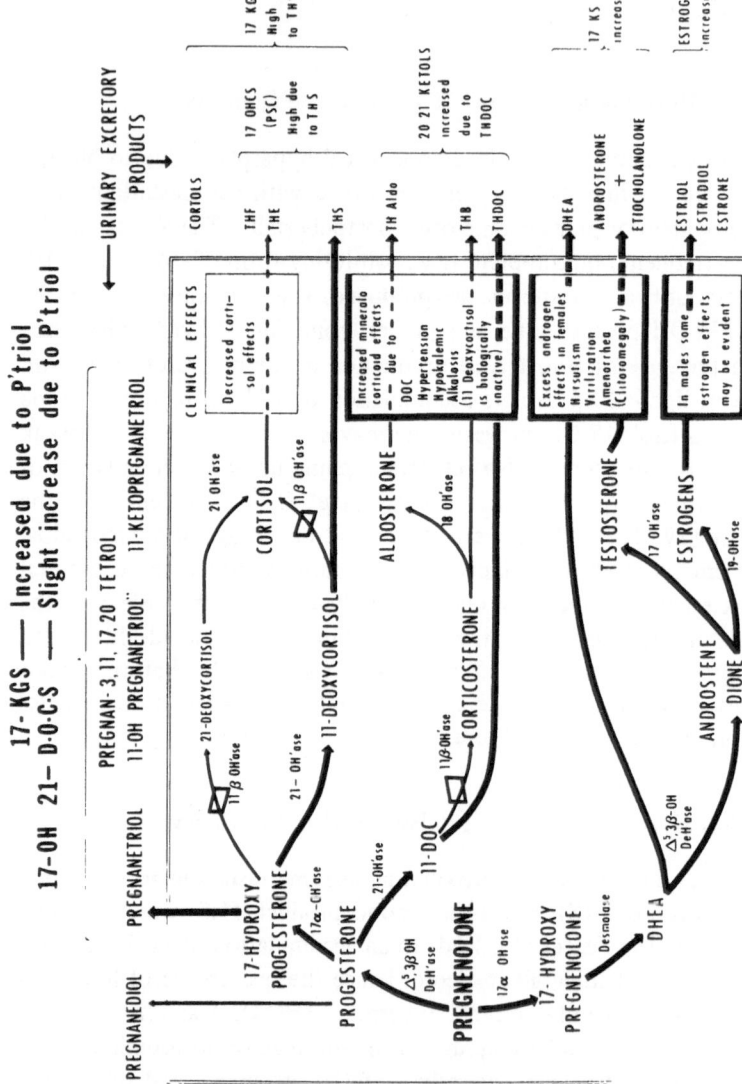

Figure 10.4. Clinical features and pattern of corticosteroid metabolites in adrenocortical 11β-hydroxylase deficiency. Clinical features are presented in the small boxes and urinary end-products are depicted outside the double-lined rectangles. (Reprinted with permission: Bacchus, 1972.)

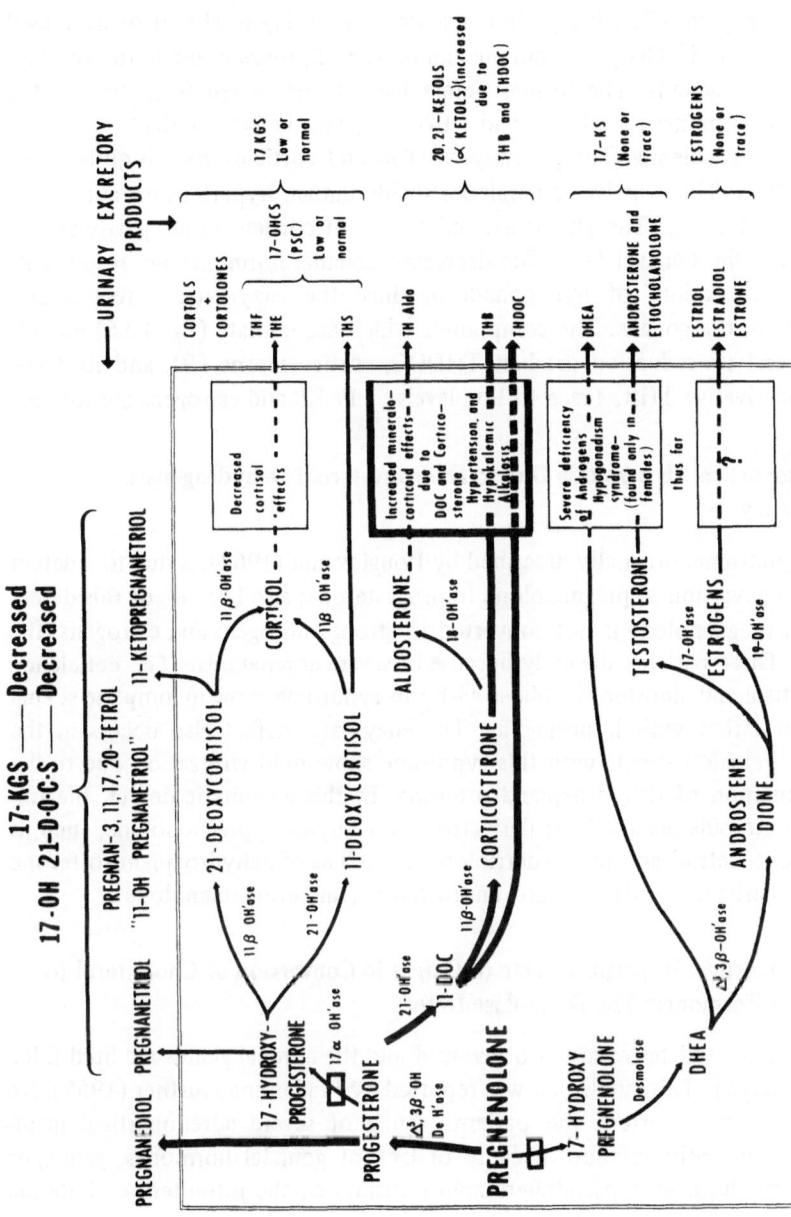

Figure 10.5. Clinical features and pattern of corticosteroid metabolites in adrenocortical 17α-hydroxylase deficiency. Clinical features are listed in the small rectangular boxes and urinary end-products are depicted outside the double-lined large rectangle. (Reprinted with permission: Bacchus, 1972.)

Adrenocortical Hyperplasia Due to 17-αHydroxylase Deficiency

This syndrome first described by Biglieri, Herron, and Brust (1966) is due to a deficiency in 17-hydroxylation reactions, resulting in absent or decreased formation of 17-OH pregnenolone and of 17-OH progesterone in the adrenals and in the gonads. The former defect leads to decreased formation of the gonadal hormones (androgens and estrogens), and the latter defect is the basis of hypocortisolemia. The pathway to DOC and corticosterone is quite active (fig. 10.5). These active mineralocorticoids induce hypertension and hypokalemic alkalosis. The glucocorticoid action of corticosterone partly substitutes for the cortisol lack. The decreased gonadal hormones are responsible for manifestations of hypogonadism, since the enzymatic defect is also present in the gonads. The compounds which accumulate (fig. 10.5) include DOC and its reduction product THDOC, corticosterone (B), and its tetrahydroderivative THB. Trace to low levels of 17-KS and estrogens are formed.

Adrenocortical Hyperplasia Due to Hydroxysteroid Dehydrogenase Deficiency

This syndrome, originally described by Bongiovanni (1962), is due to a defect in the conversion of pregnenolone to progesterone; also because of this defect 17-OH pregnenolone is not converted to strong androgens and estrogens (fig. 10.6). These patients die early because of severe adrenal crisis, *i.e.*, deficiency in cortisol and aldosterone. Males with this syndrome show incomplete sexual differentiation with hypospadias. The enzymatic defect also occurs in the testes. Female patients with this syndrome show mild virilization due to the accumulation of dehydroepiandrosterone. In this enzymatic defect, the following steroids accumulate: derivatives of 17-hydroxypregnenolone, such as Δ^5 pregnenetriol and pregnenetriolone, as well as of dehydroepiandrosterone and its derivatives, DHA sulfate, androsterone, and etiocholanolone.

Adrenocortical Hyperplasia Due to Defect in Conversion of Cholesterol to Steroid Hormones: The Desmolase Defect

The ovaries and testes are also involved and the adrenal glands are lipid-filled and enlarged. This syndrome was reported by Prader and Gurtner (1955). No survivals are reported, the patients dying of severe adrenocortical insufficiency in early infancy. Because of lack of gonadal hormones, genotype males are born with pseudohermaphroditism, *i.e.*, the intrauterine Müllerian duct system persists indefinitely.

Adrenocortical Hyperplasia Due to 18-α-Hydroxylase Defect

An 18-hydroxylase deficiency with decreased aldosterone production and salt loss has been reported. The syndrome is not fully characterized. A defect in

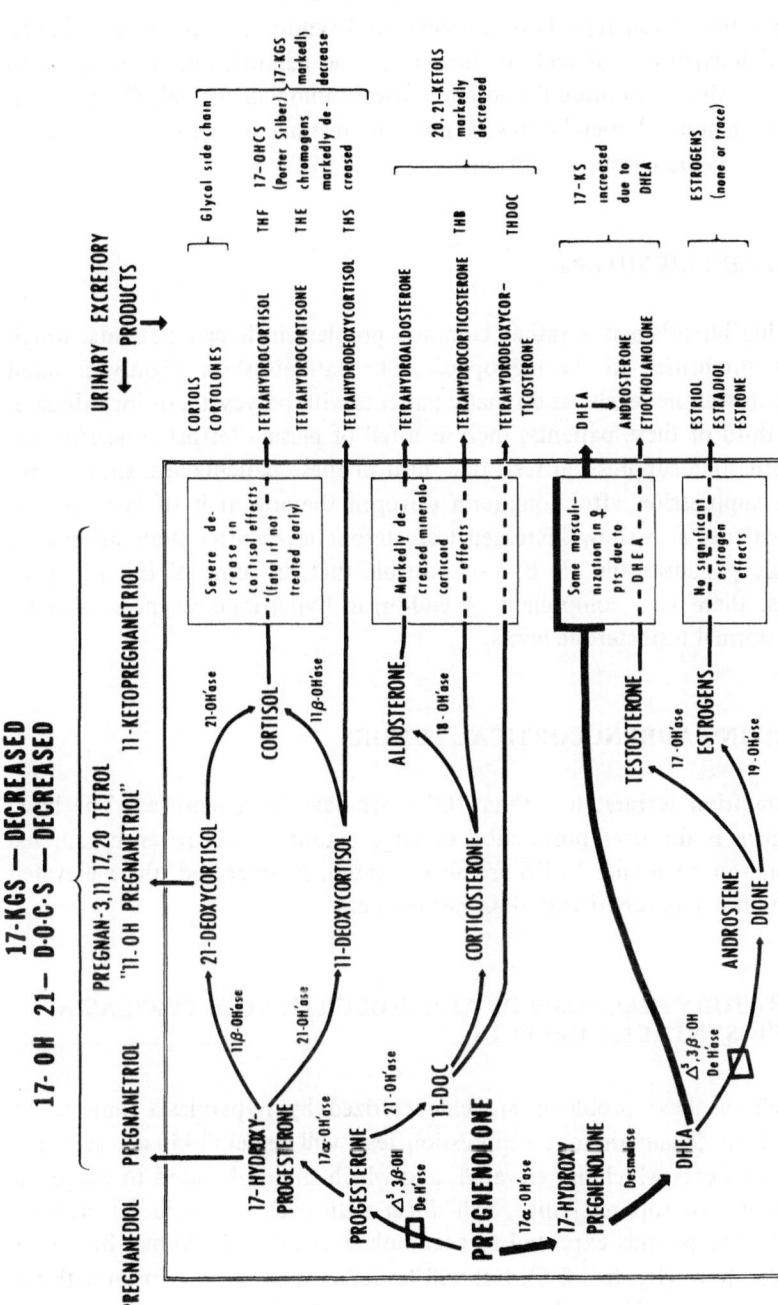

Figure 10.6. Clinical features and pattern of corticosteroid metabolites in adrenocortical Δ^5, 3β-ol dehydrogenase (HSD) deficiency. Clinical features are listed in the small rectangles and urinary end-products are outside the double-lined rectangle. (Reprinted with permission: Bacchus, 1972.)

18-hydroxydehydrogenase with elevated levels of 18-hydroxycorticosterone has been reported in one patient with excess salt loss.

There have been reports of adrenogenital syndromes presumably due to acquired biosynthetic defects in tumors of the adrenal. Diagnosis and procedures are similar to those for adrenocortical tumors in general. The accumulation of abnormal metabolites is not suppressible by exogenous corticosteroids in the neoplastic conditions.

IDIOPATHIC HIRSUTISM

Idiopathic hirsutism is a rather common problem in female patients, which may be intensified in the menopause. The patients show slightly elevated urine testosterone levels, as do many patients with polycystic ovarian disease. In one-third of these patients, there is a fall of plasma testosterone after the dexamethasone suppression test; one-third of these patients also show testosterone suppression after long-term estrogen therapy; it is of interest that these patients also show increased testosterone levels after stimulation with chorionic gonadotropin. It is also possible that, in some of this group of patients, there is a component of end-organ hyperresponsiveness to endogenous normal testosterone levels.

FEMINIZING ADRENOCORTICAL TUMORS

This condition is rare; less than 100 cases have been reported. The basic mechanism is the over production of large amounts of estrogen by adrenal carcinoma or adenoma; 17-KS are also elevated. As expected, these elevated levels are not suppressed with dexamethasone.

LABORATORY DIAGNOSIS OF ADRENOCORTICAL HYPERPLASIA WITH BIOSYNTHETIC DEFECTS

Since all of these problems are characterized by hyperplasia induced by ACTH, then dexamethasone suppression tests will be helpful in all cases. The steroid products which are elevated, and which should be used to gauge the effectiveness of suppressibility, will differ with each synthetic defect, however. The compounds expected to accumulate in these syndromes have been discussed above (fig. 8.1–8.6), but will be referred to in connection with the specific problems. The 17-KS are elevated in the C 21 hydroxylase deficiency and 11β-hydroxylase deficiency and, therefore, the 17-KS levels may be used to monitor suppressibility with dexamethasone. In a patient with virilization, hypertension, and hypokalemic alkalosis, an elevated 17-KS suppressible by dexamethasone would strongly suggest 11β-hydroxylase deficiency. Similarly, in a patient with virilization, without hypermineralocorticoidism, an elevated 17-KS suppressible by dexamethasone would be consistent with 21-hydroxylase deficiency. Specific identification of metabolites characteristic of the biosynthetic defect is possible and recommended. Studies on 17-KS excretion will not be particularly helpful in the identification of a defect in 17-hydroxylation, as 17-KS should be decreased in this condition. An increase in 17-KS in Δ^5, 3β-ol dehydrogenase deficiency, reflecting increased levels of dehydroepiandrosterone, androsterone, and etiocholanolone, may be helpful in suppression studies in that defect.

Specific Identification of the Defects

In the presence of C 21 hydroxylase deficiency, the metabolites found in excess are pregnanetriol, 17-hydroxypregnanolone, and, occasionally, 11-ketopregnanetriol. In the presence of 21 hydroxylase deficiency, these values increase to 10–70 mg, 10–20 mg, and 5 mg/24 hr respectively. The entire group of these compounds may be quantitated by a method for total 17-OH, 21 deoxycorticosteroids (Bacchus, 1972). This value is normally 0.8–3.0 mg/24 hr; in CAH, the values are increased by 10-fold or more; in the postpubertal form of this disorder, the levels are increased 3 to 5-fold.

In C 11 hydroxylase deficiency, the following compounds, in addition to 17-KS, are found in increased amounts in the urine: THS and its C 20 reduced derivative pregnan 3, 17, 20, 21 tetrol, as well as THDOC. The elevated THS and THDOC levels characteristic of 11β-hydroxylase deficiency are suppressible with dexamethasone, which also is used in the therapy of this condition.

In the presence of 17α-hydroxylase deficiency, the major compounds found in large amounts in the urine are THB and THDOC. The elevated levels of THB and THDOC are suppressible by dexamethasone.

When there is a defect in Δ^5, 3β-ol dehydrogenase, transformations along the corticosterone or the cortisol series are not possible to any significant extent. Therefore, the compounds which accumulate include Δ^5 pregnentriol and Δ^5 pregnanetriolone.

Treatment Of Adrenal Hyperplasia Due to Biosynthetic Defects

The common feature in all of the defects in nonneoplastic glands is excessive production of ACTH in response to decreased cortisol suppression of CRF (and ACTH). In 17α-hydroxylase deficiency, the component of hypogonadal manifestations is added because this defect is also present in the gonads.

The basic therapy in all forms of these biosynthetic defects is administration of doses of dexamethasone sufficient to suppress the excess ACTH release. Dosages of 0.5 mg (to 0.75 mg rarely) of dexamethasone, preferably given at bedtime, quite adequately suppress the excess ACTH. Success in this goal is readily monitored by quantitation of urinary 17-KS or of the pathognomonic end-products in the urine. Suppression to normal or low levels reflects adequate dosages of desamethasone.

The hypogonadal manifestations in 17α-hydroxylase deficiency should be treated with the appropriate gonadal hormone replacement (estrogens).

SUMMARY OF DIAGNOSTIC PROCEDURES

The clinical features of disorders of the adrenal cortex are described in the context of the biogenesis and biologic activities of adrenocortical steroid hormones. The procedures for clinical investigation of the adrenal cortex and the pituitary adrenal axis are also presented.

The following clinical laboratory tests for steroid metabolites are recommended in the diagnosis of adrenocortical disorders. These procedures are described in detail in another publication (Bacchus, 1972). In suspected adrenocortical hypofunction, when the patient is in shock, the plasma cortisol level, which should be elevated in shock due to nonadrenocortical disorders, is determined. After recovery, maintain the patient on dexamathasone (2 mg/day) and fluorocortisol (0.1 mg/day) and perform plasma cortisol studies before and after intravenous infusion of cosyntropin (0.25 mg i.v.).

When patients are not in shock, after obtaining an abnormal water diuresis test, plasma cortisol levels are determined before and after the intravenous injection of cosyntropin. The absence of an increase in plasma cortisol after a single cosyntropin challenge would be consistent with adrenocortical insufficiency. This study would be supplemented by repeat challenges with cosyntropin (every 60 min for 3 doses); if the adrenal hypofunction is secondary to pituitary disease, progressive increments in plasma cortisol levels are noted after each successive infusion of cosyntropin. An alternative, but more cumbersome, procedure involves urinary steroid response to a single 8-hr ACTH challenge. In a suspected pituitary hypofunction, repetitive (3 days) 8-hr ACTH tests are performed.

The levels of plasma cortisol before and after the intramuscular injection of 10 units of vasopressin will establish the integrity of the pituitary adrenocortical axis. Plasma cortisol after a hypoglycemia challenge provides similar information. An alternative procedure is to study the levels of plasma or urinary 11-deoxycortisol or THS respectively, before and after the administration of metyrapone.

In suspected adrenocortical hyperfunction, the following clinical laboratory steroid tests are recommended. First, plasma cortisol levels at 8:00 A.M.

and 5:00 P.M. should be taken. High levels without a circadian variation are compatible with hypercortisolemia. Second, plasma cortisol levels after overnight dexamethasone suppression test should be taken. A value of plasma cortisol 10 μg/100 ml or greater than one-half of the previous 8:00 A.M. specimen would be consistent with Cushing's syndrome. Finally, these tests may be supplemented by the more cumbersome methods for measurement of urinary steroids before and after dexamethasone suppression.

In suspected biosynthetic defects in the adrenal, determination of plasma cortisol levels at 8:00 A.M. and 5:00 P.M. should be made. These values may be lower than normal in adrenal biosynthetic defects. High levels of plasma 11-deoxycortisol are consistent with, or diagnostic of, 11β-hydroxylase deficiency. Urinary 17-OH, 21-DOCS levels in baseline 24-hr urine, and after 3 days of dexamethasone suppression should be determined. The above urine samples should also be screened for pregnanetriols and for THS. Elevation of pregnanetriols, with subsequent suppression, would be consistent with adrenal 21-hydroxylase deficiency. Elevation of THS, with subsequent suppression with dexamethasone, would be consistent with adrenal 11-hydroxylase deficiency. Elevated DOC, corticosterone, THDOC, or THB would be consistent with 17-hydroxylase deficiency. Elevated 17-KS, in the absence of increased levels of THS and along with increased levels of pregnenetriols in the urine, would be compatible with Δ^5, 3β-ol dehydrogenase (3-hydroxysteroid dehydrogenase) deficiency.

REFERENCES

Bacchus, H. 1972. Endocrine profiles in the clinical laboratory. *In* M. Stefanini (ed.), Progress in Clinical Pathology, Vol. IV. Grune & Stratton, Inc. New York, pp. 1–101.

Baxter, J. D., and P. H. Forsham. 1972. Tissue effects of glucocorticoids. Am. J. Med. 53:573–590.

Biglieri, E. G., A. M. Herron, and N. Brust. 1966. 17α-Hydroxylation deficiency in man. J. Clin. Invest. 45:1946–1954.

Bondy, P. K. 1969. The adrenal cortex. *In* Diseases of Metabolism, pp. 827–855. W. B. Saunders Company, Philadelphia.

Bongiovanni, A. M. 1962. The adrenogenital syndrome with deficiency of hydroxysteroid dehydrogenase. J. Clin. Invest. 41:2086–2092.

Conn, J. W. 1965. Hypertension, the potassium ion and impaired carbohydrate tolerande. New England J. Med. 273: 1135–1143.

Conn, J. W. 1955. Primary aldosteronism, a new clinical entity. J. Lab. & Clin. Med. 45:3–17.

Davis, W. W., and L. D. Garren. 1966. Evidence for the stimulation by adrenocorticotropic hormone of the conversion of cholesterol esters to cholesterol in the adrenal *in vitro*. Biochem. Biophys. Res. Comm. 24:805–810.

Feldman, D., J. W. Fundar, and I. S. Edelman. 1972. Subcellular mechanisms in the action of adrenal steroids. Am. J. Med. 53:545–560.

Forsham, P. H. 1969. The adrenal cortex. *In* R. H. Williams (ed.), Textbook of Endocrinology, pp. 287–379. W. B. Saunders Company, Philadelphia.

Katz, F. H., M. Lipman, A. G. Frantz, and J. W. Jailer, 1962. The physiological significance of 6β hydroxycortisol in human corticoid metabolism. J. Clin. Endocrinol. 22:71–77.

Prader, A., and Gurtner, H. P. 1955. Das syndrome des pseudohermaphroditismus masculinus. Helvet. Paediat. Acta 10:397–412.

Rovner, D. R. 1972. The enigma of idiopathic cyclic edema. Hospital Pract. 4:105–110.

Ulstrom, R. A., G. Collie, J. Burley, and R. Gunville. 1960. Adrenocortical steroid metabolism in newborn infants. II. Urinary excretion of 6-hydroxy-cortisol and other polar metabolites. 20:1080–1094.

11

Special Topics

DISORDERS OF CARBOHYDRATE METABOLISM

Several clinical disorders with gynecologic manifestations may influence the intermediary metabolism of carbohydrates. Several hormones in female endocrinology may indirectly influence carbohydrate economy and others specifically may increase the process of gluconeogenesis. Among the indirect hormonal influences on carbohydrate economy are estrogens and progesterone. There are several lines of evidence to indicate that elevated levels of estrogens may contribute to carbohydrate intolerance and an abnormal glucose tolerance curve. The lack of estrogens *per se* is not known to be associated with the opposite changes in carbohydrate kinetics, namely hypoglycemia. Disorders with major gynecologic manifestations, which are associated with decreased blood glucose levels and often with hypoglycemia, are panhypopituitarism, Sheehan's syndrome, Simmond's disease, anorexia nervosa, hypothyroidism, and adrenocortical insufficiency in its various forms. In all of the disorders except hypothyroidism and anorexia nervosa, the major mechanism for lowered glucose levels is a decrease in gluconeogenesis. The mechanism in hypothyroidism is mainly one of slow carbohydrate absorption in the duodenum, a phenomenon which is also seen in hypopituitarism and adrenocortical insufficiency. In anorexia nervosa, the altered carbohydrate metabolism is due to inanition. Neoplastic disorders with gynecologic manifestations may influence carbohydrate metabolism by destruction of the adrenals or other endocrine glands listed above by metastatic spread.

Yet other clinical disorders with gynecologic manifestations are associated with hyperglycemia and impaired carbohydrate tolerance. Prominent among these is acromegaly, whereby the increased levels of growth hormone exert an anti-insulin effect and also increase gluconeogenesis. Cushings' syndrome, whether due to hyperplasia, adenoma, or carcinoma, affects carbohydrate metabolism by increasing gluconeogenesis due to the hypercortisolemia characteristics of this syndrome. Hyperthyroidism, which may have gynecologic manifestations, alters intermediary carbohydrate metabolism by increasing both the rates of intestinal absorption of carbohydrates and of glycogenolysis. An incompletely understood carbohydrate intolerance may also be observed in the presence of various neoplasms, some of which may be originate in, or affect, the gynecologic system. These various disorders have been discussed in the appropriate sections. By far the most prevalent cause of carbohydrate intolerance in the field of gynecology and obstetrics is pregnancy. This relationship will be discussed in the aspects of the effects of pregnancy on carbohydrate metabolism and diabetes mellitus and of the effects of diabetes mellitus in pregnancy.

Carbohydrate Metabolism in Pregnancy

Several mechanisms which operate in normal pregnancy are manifested as diabetogenic factors. These factors are depicted in figure 11.1. In this diagram, the factors which influence blood glucose levels in the nonpregnant state are presented, and the effects of pregnancy superposed on this regulation are emphasized. The bulk of these are diabetogenic factors and the mechanisms of some are known. The renal threshold for glucose is variably decreased, and this may tend to lower blood glucose levels. The production of placental insulinase is well known. Insulinase produced by the liver and kidney in the nonpregnant state significantly influences the actions of insulin. For example, in the presence of chronic renal disease, a significant insulin sensitivity is partly due to the decreased levels of renal insulinase and diminished insulin degradation. In the pregnant state, placental insulinase may decrease the circulating levels of insulin. Insulinase levels are not significantly elevated in the first trimester. Late in pregnancy with placental aging, as well as at the time of delivery and removal of the placenta, the degradation of insulin is decreased because of decreased insulinase levels.

Placental production of somatomammotropin or placental lactogenic hormone is well known. This hormone exerts many of the metabolic actions of growth hormone, such as an anti-insulin action and a stimulation of gluconeogenesis. Plasma levels of cortisol are elevated in pregnancy, but this is probably due to the estrogen-induced increase in cortisol-binding globulin. High progesterone levels in pregnancy may displace cortisol from CBG, and this may result in higher circulating levels of free cortisol, with increased gluconeogenesis resulting. The participation of placental thyrotropic hormone in activating maternal thyroid activity should also be considered as a possible diabetogenic factor in pregnancy.

A quantitatively very important diabetogenic factor is the "fasting metabolism state" which occurs in pregnancy. Several biochemical parameters suggest that there is a loss of essential intermediary metabolites to the developing fetus, inducing a "fasting metabolism state" in the maternal

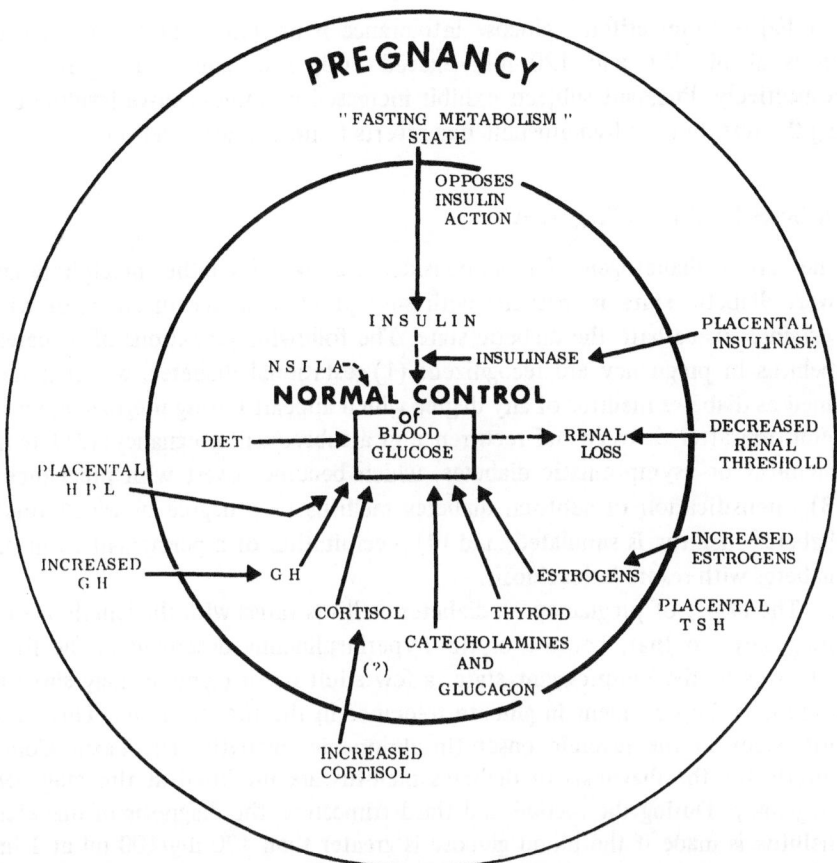

Figure 11.1. Diabetogenic factors in pregnancy. The factors which control blood glucose levels in the normal subject are presented in the center of the diagram. A positive relationship (correlation) is indicated by *solid arrows,* and inverse factors by *broken arrows.* The diabetogenic factors of pregnancy are depicted in the *outer circle* as imposed on normal control.

compartment. There is increased lipolysis in pregnancy with detectably elevated levels of free fatty acids and ketone bodies in the maternal circulation. Both factors are strongly anti-insulin; hence there is decreased insulin effect at the various target cells, *e.g.,* adipose cells and muscles. Hence, relative insulin resistance is seen in normal pregnancy.

The various factors listed above are responsible for laboratory evidence of glucose intolerance in pregnancy to different extents. The renal threshold alterations may occur quite early in pregnancy, but overt glucose intolerance is not apparent until late in the second trimester and the third trimester. Accordingly, the glucose tolerance test is essentially normal in the first trimester. The standard criteria for interpretation of the GTT at this time are identical to those for the nonpregnant state. According to the very convenient Fajans-Conn criteria, glucose intolerance is present if the blood glucose levels at 60, 90, and 120 min exceed 160, 140, and 120 mg/100 ml respectively. Pregnant subjects exhibit increased immunoreactive insulin during the test, but the hyperinsulinemia reverts to normal after delivery.

Diabetes Mellitus in Pregnancy

The various diabetogenic factors considered above may either precipitate an overt diabetic state in patients with susceptibility to the disorder, or will certainly exacerbate the diabetic state. The following gradations of diabetes mellitus in pregnancy are recognized: (1) gestational diabetes, which is defined as diabetes mellitus of any degree which appears during pregnancy, with remission after delivery and recurrence in a subsequent pregnancy; (2) latent chemical or asymptomatic diabetes, which becomes overt with pregnancy; (3) intensification of subtotal diabetes mellitus to a degree in which total diabetes mellitus is simulated; and (4) precipitation of a permanent form of diabetes with severe ketoacidosis.

The effect of pregnancy on diabetes mellitus varies with the length of the pregnancy, so that, because of the hyperinsulinemia described in the first trimester in the nonpregnant state, a few adult onset diabetics may show a temporary improvement in glucose tolerance in the first trimester. This does not occur in the juvenile onset (insulinopenic) diabetic. The Fajans-Conn criteria for the diagnosis of diabetes mellitus are modified at this stage of pregnancy. During the second and third trimesters, the diagnosis of diabetes mellitus is made if the blood glucose is greater than 170 mg/100 ml at 1 hr and greater than 120 mg/100 ml at 3 hr.

The severity of diabetes, as well as the insulin requirement, increases during the second trimester, and this continues into the third trimester. The patients may become ketosis-prone at this stage. Ketoacidosis in the pregnant individual is characterized by a moderate hyperglycemia, a marked increase in plasma ketone bodies, and a decrease in plasma CO_2. The diabetes is potentially worse in the third trimester, at which time the renal threshold for glucose may decrease further even though the sensitivity of the fetus to ketosis is now less. On the average, in view of the various factors considered above, the estimated increase in insulin requirement in the third trimester is about 66%. This may be less, however, in the presence of diabetic nephropathy. Late in the pregnancy, placental aging and delivery are associated with decreased insulin requirement. Labor is often complicated by decreased insulin requirement and hypoglycemia.

Pregnancy also influences several of the concomitants of diabetes mellitus. The susceptibility to skin and urinary tract infections is increased. Diabetic neuropathy may often get worse in pregnancy, and microvascular lesions are exacerbated so that latent nephropathy may become overt and intensified, even though this change may be temporary. Pregnancy is often associated with temporary exacerbation of diabetic retinopathy.

Effects of Diabetes Mellitus on Pregnancy   In 1882, Mathews Duncan reported that in 22 diabetic pregnancies under his care, there were 9 fetal deaths. He also pointed out that large babies are characteristic in the diabetic patients. It is now known that the tendency to produce large babies may antedate the diagnosis of diabetes by several years. However, fetal loss rate is not necessarily increased during this prodromal period, and it is not until within a 5-yr period of diagnosis that an increased fetal loss is noted. The mechanisms of large babies and diabetic embryopathy involve one or several of the following: increased growth hormone levels; genetic background; and fetal B-islet cell hyperplasia which may be secondary to hyperglycemia.

Despite the increased fetal size characteristic of diabetic pregnancies, fetal loss is confined largely to the smaller babies. Neonatal deaths of babies of diabetic pregnancies are noted within 3 days and the most frequent cause is the presence of hyaline membrane disease. Islet cell hyperplasia is also quite prevalent in such babies. The excess weight in diabetic embryopathy is due to an increase in fat and glycogen deposition, and the water content is low or normal. Other causes of high fetal loss are renal vein thrombosis and other congenital anomalies. Fetal loss rate in a worldwide series of over 4,000 diabetic pregnancies was 13.5–37%.

The most common complications of diabetes in the pregnant woman are hydramnios, toxemia, and ketoacidosis. In some series, at least 50% of diabetic pregnancies showed the presence of hydramnios; this, however, is not overtly ascribable to hyperglycemia. Severe hydramnios (volumes of 1,000–10,000 cc) are a most severe threat to the fetus. Toxemia of pregnancy was found in about 50% of diabetic pregnancies prior to 1933 but, with appropriate dietary and insulin management, this has decreased sufficiently as to be relatively unusual. In the preinsulin era, maternal dwarfism with pelvic maldevelopment was seen quite frequently in insulinopenic diabetes mellitus. There was a relative decrease in fertility in patients with diabetic dwarfism however.

Management of Pregnancy in Diabetes Mellitus   In an attempt to simplify management of diabetic pregnancies, White (1971) devised a classification of pregnant diabetes according to duration and severity. Based on this classification, fetal salvage rates have been determined. Class A pregnant diabetics are diagnosed by glucose tolerance tests only, and show no decrease in fetal salvage rate. Class B are diabetics whose onset was at over 20 yr of age and of a duration of less than 10 yr. These patients show no vascular lesions, and the fetal salvage rate is about 67%. Class C includes patients whose onset of diabetes is between ages 10–19 yr, with a duration between 10–19 yr, and lacking any vascular lesions. The fetal salvage rate in this group is 48%. Class

D includes diabetics whose onset was at less than 10 yr of age, with duration of disorder longer than 20 yr and showing vascular lesions such as retinitis and calcified vessels in the legs. The fetal salvage rate in this group is 32%. Class E diabetic pregnant patients have overt diabetes mellitus with calcified pelvic arteries. In this group the fetal salvage rate is around 13%. Class F patients exhibit overt diabetes with diabetic nephropathy. Fetal salvage rate in this group is extremely poor, around 3%. Class R patients exhibit overt diabetes mellitus with diabetic retinopathy, nephropathy, and repeated fetal loss. Other classifications, with emphasis on individualization of management, have been devised.

In milder degrees of diabetes, babies are carried to term, and delivery at less than 36 wk gestation is reserved for patients with vascular disease and nephropathy. Careful calculation of the expected date of confinement is mandatory, as premature delivery is frequently necessary. Delivery at 36 wk is the earliest stage with a reasonable chance of fetal survival. Survival rates are higher with delivery at 37 wk. It is likely that Caesarean section has no real advantages over induction except in very early deliveries.

Chemical Parameters Employed in Monitoring Diabetic Pregnancy Circulating and excretion levels of estrogens and pregnanediols are frequently employed in following the health of the fetal-placental unit (Ostergard, 1973; Spellacy and Cohn, 1973). More recently, the levels of somatomammotropin have been employed in the assessment of placental aging. Estriols and pregnanediols are both increased, especially in the third trimester. These steroids reflect synthetic activities in the fetal-placental unit. Because the production of estriol sulfate is dependent on the fetal compartment (see Chapter 4), this measurement is often employed to specifically monitor fetal health. Estriol excretion below 5 mg/24 hr or an acute drop from previously higher levels reflect defects in the compartment of the fetal-placental unit. Significant decreases in urinary pregnanediol also reflect defects in the fetal-placental unit. A normal level of pregnanediol in the face of low estriol levels indicates the presence of fetal problems. These procedures are not widely employed because of the time lapse required for 24-hr urine collections and because of relative unavailability of rapid accurate methods of quantitation of estriols and other estrogens. Some workers have suggested that the excretion of these metabolites should be correlated with urine creatinine so that random urinary collections may be employed. Availability of plasma levels of these metabolites by radioimmunoassay and competitive protein-binding methods should permit wider utilization of these methods of fetal-placental monitoring. With this information, the time of termination of the pregnancy would be more safely ascertainable.

Methods of Monitoring Diabetes Mellitus in Pregnancy The practical methods of monitoring diabetic control in pregnancy include the maintenance of ideal body weight appropriate to the stage of pregnancy in the context of normoglycemia appropriate to the stage of pregnancy. The presence of glycosuria is useful only as a rough guide, but because of alterations of renal threshold in pregnancy, this measure should not be employed for regulating the dose of insulin therapy. Consistent absence of glycosuria, in view of lowered renal threshold, should be regarded as an indication of persistent hypoglycemia.

Management of Diabetes Mellitus in Pregnancy The goals in diabetic management are the prevention of acute and long-term concomitants of diabetes. The immediate goals are the maintenance of ideal body weight and normoglycemia appropriate to the stage of pregnancy. Therefore, the criteria of management are essentially similar to those in nonpregnant patients, with modifications relative to diet especially of carbohydrates because of the "fasting metabolism state" and renal threshold alterations. During the first trimester, the criteria are almost identical to those of the nonpregnant state, except for the fact that there is a slight increase in caloric requirement.

Extensive studies (Emerson, Saxena, and Poindexter, 1972) revealed that the average excess caloric expenditure during the first trimester is around 9 kcal/kg daily, and that the total daily caloric requirement for the normally active women is approximately 2,100 kcal. This increased caloric cost of pregnancy is attributable to the growth and development of the products of conception and to the altered maternal intermediary metabolism. Except in the obese or the very small women, it is likely that the diet should contain around 2,000–2,200 kcal. For small structured women, the basic dietary requirement is calculated as 1,800 kcal for the first 60 in in height and approximately 60 kcal for each additional inch of height; to this figure, a total increment of 8% is added. The desirable blood glucose levels during the first trimester should be essentially as in the nonpregnant diabetic, *i.e.*, within the Fajans-Conn criteria or up to 120 mg/100 ml 2 hr postprandially.

During the second and third trimesters, the caloric requirements in non-obese average sized pregnant women is calculated to be 2,200 kcal and 2,300 kcal, respectively. In small women, the calculation of basal requirements is employed as above, and an increment of 10–15% is added. In all cases, the total caloric intake is distributed as recommended by the American Diabetes Association, 40% carbohydrate, 40% fat, and 20% protein. The food intake should include 6,000 IU of vitamin A, 400 IU of vitamin D, 30 IU of vitamin E, and the daily requirements of thiamin, niacin, riboflavin, pyridoxine, folic acid, vitamin B12, and ascorbic acid as recommended by the National Research Council. Blood glucose levels should be maintained at around 100 mg/100 ml to less than 120 m/100 ml at 3 hr postprandially or between 140–170 mg/100 ml 1 hr postprandially. On the average, it is recommended that the patient should be permitted a total weight gain of about 12–13 kg (25–27 lb) throughout the pregnancy.

Should dietary management and exercise be inadequate in the management of diabetes in pregnancy, insulin is the recommended drug therapy. Several patients have received oral agents in diabetic management, but there are still questions as to their efficacy and teratogenic potential during pregnancy. The goal of insulin therapy along with diet is the maintenance of normoglycemia appropriate to the state of pregnancy. In this context, the desired blood glucose levels should be less than 160 mg/100 ml 1 hr postprandially and less than 120 mg/100 ml 2 hr postprandially during the first trimester. In the second and third trimesters, the desired blood glucose levels at 1 and 3 hr postprandially should be less than 170 mg/100 ml and 120/100 ml, respectively. It may occasionally be prudent to tolerate slightly higher levels than those listed in order to avoid the effects of possible hypoglycemia and consequent injury to the fetus and mother. Glycosuria is a crude guide only and should not be the basis of determining the dosage of insulin. The decreased insulin requirement just before delivery (possibly due to placental aging) prompts careful control of blood glucose at this time.

Ideal insulin therapy involves the supply of insulin appropriate to dietary challenge, so that the physiologic insulin release pattern is simulated. Because patients are often reluctant to take three injections of regular insulin daily, it is prudent to recommend a combination of regular insulin with neutral protein Hagedorn (NPH) or lente insulin before breakfast, and a similar combination prior to supper. A late evening snack of cheese and crackers is given to patients on this regimen. Best results have been obtained when two-thirds of the total daily insulin dosage is given in the morning and one-third before supper. The distribution of NPH (or lente) and regular insulins will depend on individual needs, but in general the ratio should be 3:1 to 4:1.

Management of Diabetic Ketoacidosis in Pregnancy The pathogenetic factors inducing ketoacidosis in the pregnant individual are similar to those in nonpregnant patients, except for the presence of the "fasting metabolism state" and attendant insulin resistance in pregnancy. Hyperglycemia induces as osmotic diuresis and subsequent hypovolemia and eventual oliguria. Decreased lipogenesis and increased lipolysis result in ketonemia. Mobilization of amino acids for gluconeogenesis results in increased nitrogenous compounds. Correct management requires replacement of fluid volume with normal or half-normal saline, without induction of hypo-osmolality. In the pregnant diabetic, the hyperglycemia tends to be of less severity, while the ketoacidosis is often more marked. Therefore, careful attention must be paid to the blood glucose level while insulin therapy is directed to amelioration of the ketoacidosis. Supplemental glucose is then often necessary in the course of therapy. Replacement of potassium is instituted as soon as urinary output is established. As a guideline, the typical patient in diabetic ketoacidosis has the following deficits: 6–10 L of water; 600 mEq of sodium; 400 mEq each of potassium, chloride, and bicarbonate; and 100 mEq of phosphate. Therapy should be directed to replacement of these deficits within 12–24 hr. It is essential that the blood glucose, plasma ketones, and electrolytes are monitored closely in order to ascertain need and success of therapy.

Management of Diabetes Mellitus on Day of Delivery   If the delivery is elective, the patient should be restricted from oral feedings overnight, or should be allowed only liquids. An intravenous infusion of 5% glucose in saline or water is started after the patient is given insulin by subcutaneous injection. The recommended sequence of insulin dosage is as follows: the patient receives one-half of the prepregnant dose of NPH (or lente) insulin before the intravenous glucose infusion; at the end of delivery, the remaining one-half of the prepregnant insulin requirement is given in two equal doses as regular insulin at 4- to 6-hr intervals as indicated by blood glucose levels.

CLINICAL APPLICATION OF MEASUREMENTS OF HORMONES AND THEIR DERIVATIVES

In the previous sections, references were made to several hormonal measurements in the blood and in the urine for diagnosis and followup of endocrine disorders. In this section, the most widely employed endocrine laboratory tests are listed, and their clinical applications are described. Growth hormone, TSH, FSH, LH, ACTH, prolactin, and the iodothyronines T_4 and T_3 are measured by radioimmunoassay methods; cortisol, aldosterone, deoxy-cortisol, progesterone, estradiol, estriol, and testosterone are measured by competitive protein binding or radioimmunoassay methods. The rationales of these methods have been authoritatively discussed (Odell and Daughaday, 1971). Plasma cortisol, and urinary pregnanetriol, 17-OHCS, 17-KGS, and 17-KS, among others, are measured by standard chemical methods which have been discussed *in extenso* (Bacchus, 1972).

Serum Levels of Growth Hormone

The serum levels of HGH fluctuate within a normal range throughout the day. Basal levels are increased by upright posture and activity, exercise, stress, fasting, hypoglycemia, estrogens, and L-dopa. The normal level in the child is 0–20 ng/ml and in the adult 0–10 ng/ml. In the workup of dwarfism, a level of 8–10 ng/ml effectively rules out a pituitary origin. In the workup of acromegaly, the elevated HGH levels are not suppressed by challenge of hyperglycemia.

Serum Levels of Thyroid-Stimulating Hormone

This measurement is the most sensitive test in the diagnosis of primary and secondary hypothyroidism. In the presence of low iodothyronines (T_4 and T_3), elevated TSH levels are diagnostic of primary hypothyroidism, whereas normal TSH diagnoses hypopituitary hypothyroidism. The latter is also diagnosed by the lack of a TSH elevation after TRH challenge. Hypothalamic hypothyroidism is characterized by low serum iodothyronines along with an increase of TSH to a TRH challenge. Elevated iodothyronines in the presence of TSH elevation are found in the extremely rare form of hyperthyroidism due to pituitary production of excess TSH. TSH levels are not helpful in the diagnosis of most forms of hyperthyroidism.

Serum Levels of Follicle-Stimulating Hormone

This tropic hormone is subject to wide fluctuations in adults. In women, the basal serum level is 6–30 mIU/ml, rising to 50–60 mIU at the time of the preovulatory surge. Persistent elevated FSH levels are found in the menopause and in premature ovarian senescence. Low values in postmenopausal women would be consistent with hypopituitarism. Low values are difficult to evaluate and stimulatory challenges are necessary in evaluating pituitary function. Failure of FSH to increase after FSH/LH-RH challenge diagnoses hypogonadotropinism. An increase in FSH after FSH/LH-RH, but not after clomiphene, indicates hypothalamic disease.

Serum Levels of Luteinizing Hormone

The serum levels are subject to pulsatile variations within a normal range. Basal serum levels in children range from < 1–12 mIU/ml and in women from 6–30 mIU/ml, with levels reaching 150 mIU/ml at the time of the surge under control of the cyclic center of the hypothalamus. Elevated levels (30–300 mIU/ml) are found in postmenopausal women, in premature ovarian senescence, and in the Stein-Leventhal syndrome. Because of cross-reaction with HCG, persistently elevated levels over 30 mIU/ml would suggest pregnancy or trophoblastic neoplasm.

Low levels of LH are impossible to evaluate without appropriate challenges, so that a failure of LH to rise after a challenge with FSH/LH-RH is indicative of hypopituitarism, whereas a failure to increase in response to clomiphene in the face of a significant rise following FSH/LH-RH indicates hypothalamic disease.

Serum Levels of Adrenocorticotropic Hormone

The serum levels depend on the method of radioimmunoassay, as well as on the clinical state of the individual, as stress markedly influences the serum levels of this hormone. A circadian variation in its secretion is also well known. RIA methods indicate basal levels in the evening, ranging from 0.08–0.12 mU/100 ml, and in the morning from 0.15–0.45 mU/100 ml. ACTH levels are increased in adrenocortical insufficiency, Cushing's disease, Nelson's syndrome (pituitary tumors after adrenalectomy), in congenital adrenocortical hyperplasia with biosynthetic defects, and in ACTH-secreting neoplasms. Barely detectable levels are found in hypopituitarism. Low serum ACTH levels in the presence of low cortisol would be consistent with hypopituitary hypocorticism (hypoadrenocorticotropinism). Elevated ACTH in the face of low plasma cortisol is the pattern in primary adrenal insufficiency.

Serum Levels of Prolactin

The mean plasma level of prolactin in woman is around 90 ng/ml, without any variations during the menstrual cycle. The levels increase progressively in pregnancy, reaching levels up to 300 ng/ml in the third trimester. The patterns of change with lactation were described in Chapter 8. Elevated levels (barring pregnancy) are found in the inappropriate lactation syndromes, after certain drugs, and after TRH challenge (see Chapter 8). Some studies suggest that PRL elevations are present in patients with pituitary neoplasm, and suggest its use in screening for such processes.

Serum Levels of Thyroxine

Normal serum values of this iodothyronine hormone range from 5–13 μg/100 ml. The value of total throxine should be corrected for the factor of thyroxine-binding globulin (TBG), as there are several clinical states as well as drugs which influence the levels and binding to TBG. Formulas for estimating a thyroxine index were presented in Chapter 9. Elevated values of T_4 are found in hyperthyroidism, pregnancy, early liver disease, and after estrogens. The adjusted T_4 (corrected by TBG assessment) is elevated in hyperthyroidism, but not in the other situations listed above. Elevated adjusted T_4 levels are highly reliable in the diagnosis of hyperthyroidism, but low adjusted T_4 levels are not as reliable in the diagnosis of hypothyroidism.

The free T_4 level is derived after a tedious procedure. Normal values are 1.5–4.0 ng/100 ml. The method is quite reliable in diagnosis of hyperthyroidism, and less so in hypothyroidism.

Serum Levels of Triiodothyronine

The iodothyronine hormone T_3 is biologically three to four times as potent as T_4. Circulating levels in normal subjects range from 80–220 ng/100 ml. T_3 values are elevated in hyperthyroidism, often earlier than an elevation of T_4 occurs. The entity T_3-toxicosis, which is a form of hyperthyroidism, without T_4 elevations is characterized by elevated T_3 levels, and is considered to represent an early manifestation of hyperthyroidism. T_3 levels are also elevated during antithyroid drug therapy for hyperthyroidism, as well as in the early phases of recurrent hyperthyroidism.

Plasma or Serum Levels of Cortisol

Plasma cortisol levels undergo a circadian variation with normal levels of 5–25 μg/100 ml at 8 A.M. and 2.5–12.5 μg/100 ml at 5 P.M. In Cushing's syndrome, the levels are above 30 μg/100 ml and fail to show a circadian variation. Nonsuppressibility with dexamethasone is consistent with Cushing's syndrome. Low levels are difficult to evaluate without resort to an appropriate challenge. A failure of significant elevation after a cosyntropin challenge is found in primary adrenal insufficiency. Lack of a significant elevation after a hypoglycemic challenge, in the face of an elevation after cosyntropin, is indicative of hypocorticotropinism (Chapter 10).

Plasma Levels of Estradiol

The plasma levels of estradiol vary with the phases of the menstrual cycle. During the early follicular phase, the value is around 0.006 μg/100 ml, rising to around 0.07 μg/100 ml in the late follicular phase, and decreasing to around 0.02 μg/100 ml in the midluteal phase. The values increase progressively during pregnancy. The values are extremely difficult to evaluate without associated data on FSH and LH, as well as target organ responses (see Chapter 4).

Serum Levels of Estriol

Estriol is the degradation product of estradiol and possesses weak estrogenic potency. This product is formed in the placenta from precursors provided by the fetal unit (see Chapter 4). Normal serum values in the third trimester range from 7–20 μg/100 ml. A drop in this value in the face of normal progesterone (for the stage of pregnancy) is reflection of a fetal defect. A drop in both products suggests a placental or combined placental-fetal defect.

Serum Levels of Progesterone

The serum levels of this hormone vary markedly during the menstrual cycle. In the follicular phase, the serum levels are less than 100 ng/100 ml, and are probably derived from the adrenal cortex. After ovulation and corpus luteum formation, i.e., in the luteal phase, the serum level of progesterone is around 400 ng/100 ml or above. In pregnancy, the value exceeds 800 ng/100 ml. Elevated levels of progesterone are found in 17α-hydroxylase deficiency, and are suppressible by dexamethasone.

Plasma Levels of Testosterone

Plasma testosterone values in the prepubertal female are usually less than 20 ng/100 ml, and in the adult female less than 80 ng/100 ml. This hormone is elevated to around 120 ng/100 ml in women with idiopathic hirsutism. Virilization is found in patients with values around 200 ng/100 ml. Suppression of elevated values by dexamethasone (2 mg/day) suggests an adrenocortical source of the androgen, but this concept has been challenged recently (see Chapters 6 and 10). Failure of suppression suggests an autonomous adrenal or ovarian tumor. Elevated levels are also found in the Stein-Leventhal syndrome, and this finding, in combination with normal FSH and inappropriately elevated LH, is regarded as characteristic of the syndrome.

Serum Levels of Aldosterone

The serum levels of this mineralocorticoid hormone are subject to variations due to posture, salt intake, and activity. Normal values in a patient on an adequate sodium intake (6 gm of NaCl/day) are as follows: in the supine position, 1–8 ng/100 ml and, in the upright position, 5–25 ng/100 ml. In a patient on a low sodium diet the values increase 2- to 5-fold. Normal subjects given an exogenous mineralocorticoid (9α-fluorocortisol or desoxycorticosterone) show decreased levels of serum aldosterone to less than 3 ng/100 ml. In primary aldosteronism, the elevated levels are not suppressed by exogenous mineralocorticoid administration (see Chapter 10).

Serum Levels of Deoxycortisol

Basal levels of this intermediate in adrenal hormone synthesis are less than 1 ng/100 ml of serum. These values are elevated in the adrenal biosynthetic defect in 11β-hydroxylase deficiency, as well as following the infusion or ingestion of the synthetic 11β-hydroxylase inhibitor metyrapone. The ability of the drug to inhibit the synthesis of cortisol is employed in tests to assay pituitary adrenal feedback mechanisms. Normal individuals challenged with metyrapone exhibit serum deoxycortisol levels of greater than 10 ng/100 ml. Patients with Cushing's syndrome due to hyperplasia show an exaggerated elevation, whereas patients with adrenal tumor as basis of Cushing's syndrome exhibit no change after metyrapone. This challenge is not widely used now in the diagnosis of pituitary adrenocorticotropic insufficiency.

Urine Pregnanetriol Levels

This compound is an end-product of 17-OH progesterone and is elevated in disorders associated as absolute or relative defect in 21-hydroxylation in the adrenal cortex. Normal urine levels range between 1.5–2.6 mg/24 hr. In virilizing adrenocortical hyperplasia due to 21-hydroxylase deficiency, the values may increase 20- to 30-fold, but are readily suppressible with exogenous glucocosticoid therapy. Urinary pregnanetriol may be moderately elevated in Cushing's syndrome.

Urine Tetrahydro-11-Deoxycortisol

This compound is a reduction product of the intermediate deoxycortisol. Normal values amount to less than 0.2 mg/24 hr, but may be increased very markedly (50- to 100-fold) in adrenal hyperplasia due to 11β-hydroxylase deficiency, the hypertensive form of virilizing adrenal hyperplasia (see Chapter 10). These elevated values are suppressible by exogenous glucocorticoids in this disorder. Urine levels of THS may be employed to assess pituitary adrenal dynamics after metyrapone as described above.

Urine 17-Hydroxycorticosteroids

Urinary excretion of this group of compounds is a measure of production of steroids with the 17-OH, 20, 21-ketol side chain which is present in cortisol, cortisone, and deoxycortisol. These steroids are reduced to tetrahydro derivatives prior to conjugation for urinary excretion. Normal urinary excretion of 17 OHCS is 2.5–8.4 mg/24 hr. These values are increased in Cushing's syndrome due to adenoma, carcinoma, or hyperplasia. Appropriate suppression tests were described in Chapter 10. Low levels *per se* should not be employed to diagnose adrenal insufficiency, and an ACTH challenge is necessary to determine adrenal responsiveness as reflected by elevated 17-OHCS after the challenge. In 11β-hydroxylase deficiency in hypertensive virilizing adrenal hyperplasia, the 17-OHCS elevation is due to increased production of 11-deoxycortisol, and these levels are suppressible with exogenous glucocorticoids.

Urinary 17-Ketogenic Steroids

Compounds constituting the 17-KGS include steroids with the following side chains: (1) 17-OH, 20, 21-ketol side chain as in cortisol, cortisone, and 11-deoxycortisol. (2) 17, 20, 21-glycol side chain as in cortol, cortolone, and the 20-reduced end-products of 11-deoxycortisol. (3) 17-OH, 21-deoxycorticosteroids as in 17-hydroxyprogesterone; and (4) 17-OH, 20-OH, 21-deoxy compounds as the 20α- or β-reduced end-products of 17-hydroxyprogesterone.

Normal excretion of 17-KGS in women is 7–17 mg/24 hr. These values are elevated in Cushing's syndrome, in C 21-hydroxylase and 11β-hydroxylase defects in the adrenals. (See Chapter 10 for definitive workup of elevated 17-KGS.) Urinary 17-KGS may be decreased in adrenocortical insufficiency and hypopituitarism, but definitive diagnosis requires appropriate ACTH and hypoglycemia challenges to differentiate these entities.

Urinary 17-Ketosteroids

The urinary 17-KS are derived from breakdown products of adrenal hormones, C 19 biosynthetic intermediates in testicular and ovarian hormone synthesis, and, to a small extent, from degradation of testosterone. Normal excretion in the adult female is 7–15 mg/24 hr. These values are elevated in Cushing's syndrome, as well as in adrenocortical biosynthetic defects such as 21-hydroxylase deficiency, 11β-hydroxylase deficiency, and hydroxysteroid dehydrogenase deficiency (see Chapter 10). In these synthetic defects, exogenous glucocorticoid therapy is followed by suppression. Certain ovarian tumors may be associated with increased 17-KS (see Chapter 6). Low levels are found in adrenocortical deficiency, but appropriate challenges are necessary to establish the diagnosis.

REFERENCES

Bacchus, H. 1972. Endocrine profiles in the clinical laboratory. *In* M. Stefanini (ed.), Progress in Clinical Pathology, pp. 1–10. Grune & Stratton, Inc., New York.
Emerson, K., B. Saxena, and E. L. Poindexter. 1972. Caloric cost of normal pregnancy. Obst. & Gynec. 40:786–791.
Odell, W. D., and W. H. Daughaday, (eds.) 1971. Principles of Competitive Protein-Binding Assays. J. B. Lippincott Company, Philadelphia.
Ostergard, D. R. 1973. Estriol in pregnancy. Obst. & Gynec. Surv. 28:215–231.
Spellacy, W. N., and J. E. Cohn. 1973. Human placental lactogen levels and daily insulin requirements in patients with diabetes mellitus complicating pregnancy. Obst. & Gynec. 42:330–333.
White P. 1971. Pregnancy and diabetes. *In* A. Marble et al. (eds.), Joslin's Diabetes Mellitus, pp. 581–598. Lea & Febiger, Philadelphia.

Index